More Praise for *Med School*

"*Med School* is a fascinating look at medical school life in the fifties and clearly shows us how far medicine has come in the last half century. The history, the people, and the wonderful writing style hooked me right away and never let me go until the very end . . . and I still wanted more. Great read for anyone interested in medicine and its history."

KEVIN SODEN, M.D.
Author of *The Art of Medicine: What Every Doctor and Patient Should Know*

"A wonderful collection of vignettes from the author's experience as a medical student, laden with descriptions of faculty idiosyncrasies, humor, student escapades, and cogent observations on medical practice and its practitioners."   **ROSCOE. R. ROBINSON, M.D.**
Vice Chancellor for Health Affairs, Emeritus, Vanderbilt University

"This book is released at a time in the history of medicine when our society, litigation, and technology are forcing physicians to become shrewd businessmen and women rather than wise physicians free to love, fully appreciate, and care for their patients as Clifton Meador has done throughout his career. For those of us who treasure our medical school memories, *Med School* sends us on an exciting trip. For those just entering the world of medicine, it provides motivation and invaluable guidelines."   **BETTY RUTH SPEIR, M.D.**
Clinical Associate Professor of Obstetrics and Gynecology,
Clinical Professor of General Surgery, University of South Alabama College of Medicine

"A medical education provides both inspirational and perspirational experiences. Dr. Meador cites examples of such matters in a lively and humorous manner with accuracy and spirit. There are other books and articles about the experience of medical school; however, this treatise is most unique among such examples in that the experiences are viewed through his eyes, ears, and participation of real events. The chronicle he has presented is an altogether riveting account of happenings as a student of medicine in a particular medical school in a particular time."   **JOHN CHAPMAN, M.D.**
Dean Emeritus, School of Medicine, Vanderbilt University

"With wit and imagination, Clifton Meador has captured the rigors of medical school, the camaraderie between classmates, and the special relationship of students and faculty at Vanderbilt Medical School during the fifties."   **ERIC CHAZEN, M.D.**
Clinical Professor of Pediatrics, School of Medicine, Vanderbilt University

"I started Vanderbilt Medical School in 1948. My memory of those days is hours of studying and multiple labs. Dr. Meador's book recalls the joy of learning, and the thrill of making an accurate diagnosis by history alone. His recall of his classmates and teachers is superb! His genius of doing these many things makes this a book for all time."

BILL WADLINGTON, M.D.
Clinical Professor of Pediatrics, Vanderbilt Children's Hospital

"Dr, Meador's account of medical school in the early fifties transcends place and captures a time when science had just begun to transform the practice of medicine. Attention to what the patient said was the sharpest tool in the physician's arsenal. The process of shaping the medical doctor is told in a series of often amusing and frequently insightful stories by a naturally endowed storyteller. This collection will leave the reader with an appreciation for medicine without the hype (and expense) of modern-day technology and pharmacy."   **CHARLES F. FEDERSPIEL, PH.D.**
Professor Emeritus of Biostatistics, School of Medicine, Vanderbilt University

BOOKS BY CLIFTON K. MEADOR, M.D.

A Little Book of Doctors' Rules, by Clifton K. Meador, M.D. Philadelphia, Penn.: Hanley and Belfus, 1992.

A Little Book of Nurses' Rules, by Rosalie Hammerschmidt, R.N., and Clifton K. Meador, M.D. Philadelphia, Penn.: Hanley and Belfus, 1993.

Pearls from a Pediatric Practice I, by William Wadlington, M.D., and Clifton K. Meador, M.D. Philadelphia, Penn.: Hanley and Belfus, 1998.

A Little Book of Doctors' Rules II: A Compilation, by Clifton K. Meador, M.D. Philadelphia, Penn.: Hanley and Belfus, 1999.

A Little Book of Emergency Medicine Rules, by Corey M. Slovis, M.D., Keith D. Wrenn, M.D., and Clifton K. Meador, M.D. Philadelphia, Penn.: Hanley and Belfus, 2000.

How to Raise Healthy and Happy Children: A Pediatrician's Pearls for Parents, by William Wadlington, M.D., Clifton K. Meador, M.D., and Marietta Howington, M.A. Authors Choice Press, an imprint of iUniverse.com, Inc., 2001.

The Unknown Woman and Her Children: The Meador Family of Myrtlewood, by Clifton K. Meador, 1995.

*Translated into Japanese, Spanish, Polish, Italian, and Indonesian. German translation pending.

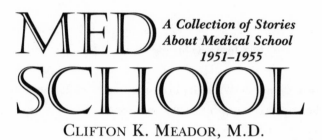

MED SCHOOL

A Collection of Stories
About Medical School
1951–1955

CLIFTON K. MEADOR, M.D.

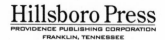

Hillsboro Press

PROVIDENCE PUBLISHING CORPORATION
FRANKLIN, TENNESSEE

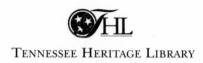

TENNESSEE HERITAGE LIBRARY

Printed in the United States of America

07   06   05   04   03   1   2   3   4   5

Library of Congress Catalog Card Number: 2003112450

ISBN: 1-57736-311-6

Cover design by John Tracy and Kelly Bainbridge

HILLSBORO PRESS
an imprint of
Providence Publishing Corporation
238 Seaboard Lane • Franklin, Tennessee 37067
www.providence-publishing.com
800-321-5692

This book is dedicated to members of the class of 1955,
to the faculty who taught us,
and to the patients
whose suffering made us better doctors.

CONTENTS

ACKNOWLEDGMENTS

MANY PEOPLE HAVE CONTRIBUTED TO THE FINAL VERSION of this book.

I want to thank Mary H. Teloh and James Thweatt of the Historical Section of the Eskind Library of Vanderbilt for their time and patience in retrieving written and photographic materials.

Michael Burgin edited some of the manuscript and offered many suggestions for improvements.

Mary Neal Meador did a careful job of editing the final manuscript.

The following people read earlier drafts of the manuscript and offered suggestions and helpful criticisms: Dr. Betty Ruth Speir, Dr. Charles Chambliss, Dr. Oscar Crofford, Dr. Jean Cortner, Dr. Ben Moore, Dr. Walter Puckett, Dr. William Wadlington, Martha Kirkpatrick Crabtree, Dr. Wallace Faulk, Dr. Robert Collins, Dr. Cathy Taylor, Dr. Diana Marver, Dr. Eric Chazen, Dr. Lewis Lefkowitz, Stephen Salisbury, Dr. Roy Elam, Martha and Pat Clark, Celine Meador, Ann Meador Shayne, Jon Shayne, Elizabeth Meador Driskill, Dr. and Mrs. Robert Sanders, Tom Blankenship, Dr. Kevin Soden, Dean Emeritus James Pittman, Dr. Harris Riley, Dr. Myron Stocking, Dean Emeritus John Chapman, and Jack Wheeler.

Virginia Fuqua-Meadows arranged my schedules and assisted in many ways in preparing the manuscript.

I want to give special thanks to my brother, Daniel J. Meador III, for his careful reading, encouragement, and strengthening sugges- tions. His son, Dan, suggested the title.

I want to thank my wife, Kathleen, for supporting my many hours of retreat. I also want to express my love and appreciation to all of my children: Clif, Aubrey, Ann, Elizabeth, Mary Kathleen, Graham, and Rebecca. The older ones made helpful suggestions, and the younger ones tolerated my time alone.

PROLOGUE

I DECIDED TO STUDY MEDICINE SHORTLY AFTER MY FIFTH birthday. I am not certain what led me to make a life decision at such an early age. Perhaps my desire stemmed from time spent observing and helping my father, a veterinarian. And I had uncles who were physicians.

Or maybe, as cliché as it may sound, an early brush with death ignited a desire to preserve life. When I was five years old, I developed lobar pneumonia with empyema—fluid in the chest cavity—and had a chest tube inserted. There were no antibiotics then, and the mortality rate of the disease was about 90 percent. I was in a coma for two weeks and in the hospital for three months. Apparently, as I would read later, a conspicuously high number of those who survive a near-fatal illness at an age younger than ten enter the healing professions. In many primitive cultures, survival of a fatal illness is an essential prerequisite to becoming a shaman.

Or maybe it was the man who cared for me during my illness more than the illness itself. Old Dr. Vastine Stabler took care of me with the pneumonia. I can still smell the ether he emitted when he came into my room on his twice-daily rounds. Dr. Tine, as we called him, graduated from Vanderbilt School of Medicine some time in the 1880s, and was as close to a saint as I have known. Whatever the reasons, I never wavered in my decision. Grammar school and high school were just pre-pre-med for me.

When I finally got there, I loved medical school. I had waited for it for nearly fifteen years, and it was a magical experience. I found the study of the human body completely absorbing. For four years, my classmates and I learned about the normal and abnormal states of man. In writing these stories, I hope to capture the zeitgeist of medicine as it was taught and practiced in the mid-twentieth century. I also want to capture some of the spirit of Vanderbilt School of Medicine as it was while rebuilding itself from the human depletions of World War II. Most of all, I want to try to tell the stories of the day-to-day experiences of going to medical school with some of my classmates from 1951 to 1955.

Here, then, are stories of some of my classmates, professors, and patients. All of them taught me for four of the most exciting years of my life. I first wrote these stories in the early 1970s, put them away, and rewrote them over the past year. All of the stories are true. Of course there is some coloration. After all, as Mark Twain points out, it is sometimes necessary to lie in order to tell the truth. While I have changed the identity of many to avoid any embarrassment, I have used the real names of my professors and a few of my classmates out of great respect and admiration.

Clifton K. Meador, M.D.
Nashville, Tennessee
July 18, 2003

General Plan of Instruction

EACH ACADEMIC YEAR WITH THE EXCEPTION OF THE FIRST (semester) is divided into three trimesters of eleven weeks each. This feature of the curriculum tends, to some extent, to break down the sharp distinction between the classes. It also allows students to return to departments in which they have developed special interests. Definite allotments of time are available in each year for elective work. There is no scheduled work on Saturday afternoon.

Although there is no sharp demarcation in the curriculum between the laboratory and the clinical courses, the first year and the greater part of the second year are taken up in the study of the medical sciences—anatomy, biological chemistry, physiology, bacteriology, pathology, and pharmacology.

Fees and Expenses

Application Fee (To accompany Application Form)......................$5.00

Tuition Fee for the Academic Year (three terms)......................$800.00

This fee is payable in equal installments, at the beginning of each term. An arrearage in tuition for any session must be paid before admission to the succeeding session.

Contingent Fee...$10.00
This fee covers breakage of apparatus and damage to buildings, and will be returned, less charges, at the close of each academic year.

Diploma Fee, charged to Graduating Students, payable during the third trimester. $5.00

Students who register for the regular courses in this Medical School must pay the full tuition each year. There will be no exception to this rule.

The average annual expenses of a student in the School of Medicine, exclusive of clothes and incidentals but including living accommodations are estimated as amounting to approximately $1200 to $1400.

Catalogue for 1951–1952
School of Medicine
Vanderbilt University

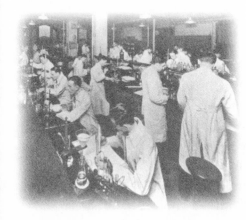

THE
LOST BOYS

Medical Fraternities: There are two medical fraternities with chapters at Vanderbilt, Alpha Kappa Kappa and Phi Chi. A large number of men enjoy the advantages of living together in these fraternity houses. They meet the same standards of inspection that are required of the University housing arrangements. Room and board in these houses is around $40 per month.

Catalogue for 1951–1952, page 60
School of Medicine
Vanderbilt University

IN SOME PLACES, THE ABSENCE OF A WOMAN'S INFLUENCE is immediately apparent. Hunting lodges. Bachelor pads. And, of course, fraternity houses. One look at the Phi Chi medical fraternity, our home-away-from-home for four years of medical school, and you knew you were looking at an estrogen-free zone.

Technically, Phi Chi was a medical fraternity, or rather, had *once* been a medical fraternity. Now it was a boarding house, overseen by no one. The previous student house manager had spent the national Phi Chi dues on a blast-out party at the end of the year. Treasury depleted, we refused to pay back the dues, and that led to our expulsion from the national organization of Phi Chi fraternities. None of us cared. All we wanted was a place to eat and sleep. We kept the Phi Chi sign over the door of the house, and the charter plaque stayed over the mantel in the living room. We figured if they really wanted to kick us out, they would have to come and remove the sign and plaque. We continued to call ourselves Phi Chis, not out of any pride, but out of habit.

We had no house mother, and even the idea of a university standard of inspection was absurd. Over the years an amorphous mass of waste and discarded junk had accumulated throughout the house. The living room had three large over-stuffed sofas, worn threadbare from years of repeated suturing practice on the fabric. Each crevice in the sofas was filled with a ground-in mixture of pages torn from old journals, surgical masks, scrub caps, pieces of scrub suits, rubber tubing, parts of stethoscopes, an occasional sock, or a T-shirt here and there. Newspapers were scattered across the floor of the room. Around the edges of the room were stacks of old issues of the *New England Journal of Medicine*, *JAMA*, and a variety of *Annals of Medicine* or *Surgery*, and other medical journals. The single bookcase was overrun with textbooks. Most of the books were long since outdated and had not been opened for years. If a party was planned, someone would push the mass of accumulated debris tightly against the walls or under the sofas and chairs. Beds were never fully made; blankets were pulled up so books and clothing would not get lost in the sheets. Clothes were put over the backs of chairs and on top of the desks.

Although fifteen of us slept and ate there, no one really lived in the house. Most of the day and late into the night, the house was completely empty. During daylight hours we were only there for lunch and supper, prepared by James Walton and his assistant cook. It was a base of operations, like an aircraft carrier, and we were all constantly on maneuvers elsewhere. No one even studied in the house. All studying and work was done at the medical school or hospital. The house was a place to sleep deeply and to eat ravenously, from which to leave early and to which to return late, before the process repeated itself the next day.

There was one exception to this regimen. On Friday nights, those of us who lived in the house showed up for supper, entertainment, and comfort.

Friday supper would usually begin with Oscar reading his mother's weekly letter. He read slowly and deliberately, never asking if we wanted to listen. Oscar just assumed we wanted him to read his mother's letters out loud. He was right. We did. We looked forward to them and felt dejected if he didn't have one, which only happened a few times. His mother was a regular writer, and those of us who got little or no mail adopted her secretly as our own mother. Oscar realized this in some unspoken way, and his sharing of her letters was his way of letting us know that he knew and understood our loneliness. He read every word with no editing. And as he did, each of us became a member of his family.

Dear Oscar,

I hope you got the new underwear I sent. I couldn't get the colors I wanted, so you will just have to wear what I could get on sale at Goldsmith's.

Oscar held up some bright red and blue boxer shorts, continuing to read the letter through his giggles.

I went up to the farm last week, and Mr. Lewis said one of the cows got caught in a mud wallow and died. He had to pull her body out with a tractor, and said it nearly tore up the tractor's rear axle to do it. Nellerine hasn't had her colt yet, but Mr. Lewis said she was doing fine.

I am sending you some brownies to share with all the boys at the house. You be sure to give each at least one a piece. Now don't go eating all of them by your-self. And don't you hide the box either. I know the boys will tell on you if you do.

I saw Jean's mother last week out shopping. She said Jean sends his laundry home in the mail just like you do, so don't think you are strange to do that. A lot of nice boys do that, otherwise they wouldn't sell those mail-it-home laundry boxes like you have. Now aren't you glad I made you take one to school with you?

Study hard and learn to be a good doctor. Write me what you are studying.

Love,
Mom

We would yell out things we wanted Oscar to write back to his mother. Questions we had about the horses or cows, and thanks for the brownies. Sometimes we suggested other foods she could send or, in our worst moods, made up obscene stories about Oscar and threatened to write her on our own. (We never did.) Every time Oscar read one of the letters, he would get as tickled as the rest of us, laughing at his mother's concerns and small worries, but obviously glowing in the love her letters showed. It was like getting our own letters from home to hear Oscar read his mail. I never realized until years later what those letters meant to me each week.

During Oscar's Friday readings, we transformed from young men who were med school students to boys who missed their families. We were the Lost Boys living in a particularly messy hideout, and Oscar's mom was our absentee Wendy.

After Oscar's reading, Wally would often take center stage. If Oscar's mother was Wendy, Wally was Peter Pan. He would tell us about the many Captain Hooks, in the form of faculty, that we would face in the classes ahead of us.

Wally had been president of the undergraduate student body before medical school—a Big Man on Campus. He was also a year ahead of us, so he had a certain credibility about him. He was loaded with charisma and entertained us with stories by the hour. The freshmen were headed into gross anatomy, so Wally, a sophomore, was giving us the scoop on the faculty and what we should expect.

Wally's basic premise was that the faculty was out to get us and would do anything to build pressure and torment us. They existed only to harass and do whatever it took to break us down so that they could fail us out of school. Better yet, they wanted to run us off, make us want to leave, make us plead to leave, do anything to get out of the misery of the horrible burden of study. This was Wally's thesis, and he was diligent in his defense of it. He was an artist in his exaggerated, even operatic, portrayal of each professor.

Our first ordeal in the ritual of medical school was gross anatomy, the course where we dissected the body of a human being. With the course came Wally's first portrayal. There were two faculty members in the anatomy department. One was Dr. Sam Clark, a refined scholar, kind, even-tempered, calm, and the picture of a gentleman. "Hell," as Wally would explain, "Dr. Sam can afford to be nice, to be quiet, because he's got the meanest son of a bitch in the world in the name of . . ." At this, Wally would pause, slide his glasses up on top of his head, push his sleeves up to his elbows, look side to side like he was about to reveal some dread secret and continue, ". . . Junnnnnnn . . . Guuullllll . . . Jimmmmmmm." His voice started low, guttural, and barely audible, before lurching up into a rasping gurgle of horror. He would never pronounce the name normally. It was always accompanied with full flourish, the glasses shifted to his head, sleeves pulled up, glancing side to side, and then the low rumbling slide into a protracted rattling of JUN-GULL-JIM.

"Just you wait until you are up to your elbows in that cadaver," he warned, "trying to find the ischio-rectal fossa, the most hidden and incomprehensible part of human anatomy, and all of a sudden JUN . . . GUL . . . JIM is there, looking over your shoulder. He appears from nowhere, making no sound whatsoever. He just appears at the table . . . and pulls that sharp metal probe out of his pocket.

"NOW, MISTER, show me the ischio-rectal fossa and demonstrate its anterior defining margin and its posterior and caudal and cephalad extensions. CAN YOU DO THAT FOR ME? . . . NOW!!!" By now Wally *was* Jungle Jim. He was standing there at the cadaver, breathing down your neck as you listened. And now, standing by the table with a knife in his hand, he would slowly begin to tap the tabletop with the tip of the knife, punctuating each word. "The" . . . tap-tap-tap . . . "ischio" . . . tap-tap-tap . . . "rectal" . . . tap-tap-tap . . . "fossa." . . . tap-tap-tap . . . "Show" . . . tap-tap-tap . . . "ME" . . . tap-tap-tap . . . "NOWWWW!" By now fully crazed, wild-eyed, and looking off into space, Wally was carried away by his performance.

By this point the upper classmen present would be laughing hysterically. We wanted to laugh too, but there was something too real, too entirely feasible about the character for us to dismiss it lightly. We knew Wally was exaggerating, but not all that much. After all, "Jungle

Jim" had been the man's nickname for years. Mild-mannered professors, kindly ones, don't get nicknames like "Jungle Jim." There had to be some truth to both the name and Wally's portrayal of him.

"Look out when the knife probe appears!" Wally warned. "Two years ago, he impaled a student's hand smack onto the thigh of a cadaver. Probe went clear through the hand . . . deep into the cadaver's leg. If he pulls that probe out of his pocket, you have made some big mistake. You are screwed if he has to go for the probe." At this, Wally collapsed into his chair, laughing. But the spell had been cast, the warning given.

The next week, after meeting Jungle Jim—or, Dr. Jim Ward, as the nonterrified called him—Oscar, Jean, and I made a solemn pact. "Our one goal," Oscar said, "is to never, never have Jungle Jim come to our table. Ever. Agree?" Jean and I nodded agreement.

Although we would never admit it and would even deny it if questioned, we loved the premise behind Wally's warning tales. We wanted medical school to be hard, tough, and nearly impossible. Each of us drew some silent, unexpressed parallel with marine boot camp or the plebe year at West Point or Annapolis. Wally was our equivalent of a "first classman," though he only hazed indirectly. With his weekly tales of terror, Wally was communicating the depth of the challenge we faced. Awareness of this challenge slowly knitted our loose fraternity of boys into a group of professionals. Together, we would endure this ordeal, and those of us who survived would become physicians and surgeons.

For all of his exaggeration and theatrics, Wally was basically correct. Nearly every professor in nearly every course instilled fear with their demands and expectations. And though failure to respect this might not result in a hand skewered by a metal probe, it could result in failing out of medical school. In his own way, Wally provided a primer that we studied to avoid the faculty's wrath and to better travel the rigorous road that lay ahead.

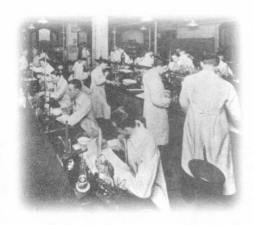

2

WEIGHTS
AND MEASURES

421. Gross Anatomy. — This course is devoted to a systematic dissection of the human body. The instruction is largely individual and the work of the student is made as independent as possible. Twenty-seven hours a week during the first semester of the first year.

422. Histology. — This course is devoted to giving the student a familiarity with the normal structure of the principal tissues and organs of the body. Fresh tissues are used wherever possible for the demonstration of normal cellular function, and students are taught the use of stains in analyzing the characteristics of particular cells. Twelve hours a week during the first trimester of the first year.

423. Neurology. — The histological aspect of the nervous system, including the structure of nerve cells, fibers and endings, the histology and pathways of the spinal cord, the structure and connections of cerebrospinal and autonomic nerves and ganglia, and the histology of the organs of special sense. Twelve hours a week for five weeks at the end of the first semester of the first year.

Catalogue for 1951–1952
School of Medicine
Vanderbilt University

IF ONE PLOTTED THE STRESS AND WORKLOAD OF FOUR years of medical school on a curve, the apogee would come just before the end of the first semester of the first year. As the final leaves drifted from tree to ground, our gross anatomy class began the study of the head and neck, by far the most complex and dreaded component of the course.

Beyond the normal strain of memorization and identification, the study of the head and neck area carries with it a degree of stress heightened by forced proximity. Tensions rise when four people gather and concentrate all their attention and activity within a four-by-four-foot cube, all trying to see and dissect at the same time. Imagine telling four people to carve a turkey at the same time, with the understanding that anyone who did not participate actively would receive nothing. To make things worse, on a cadaver the dissection of a deeper layer necessarily destroys the layer above. This was in contrast to the lower areas of the body, where the entire dissection could be laid bare, displayed, and examined thoroughly. In the most complex part of the body, we had one shot at seeing the anatomy, and then we had to move on to the deeper structures. By the time we finished, there was very little left to see except the back of the skull and the backbone.

Hank and I worked as a pair on one side of the cadaver. Oscar and Jean worked on the opposite side. We were physically tired from more than two months of daily dissection. We were emotionally drained, and had long ago submerged what was left of our spiritual selves into the study of gross anatomy. Wally had predicted that, by month's end, two of us would get in a fight. In the three years I would know Wally, this marked the only time he would be guilty of understatement. There was hardly a day that Oscar and Jean did not yell at each other, or that Hank and I did not get into a shoving contest to push the other one out of the way to get a look.

Then in the midst of the study and stress, a second course was added. Histology, the study of body tissues, carried with it demands on our memory and time nearly equal to anatomy. The treadmill had sped up considerably, and we had to run faster or fall off the back.

We coped by group study. It kept us from straying off into trivia or getting lost in too much detail. Early in the first year, Hank and I began studying together every night. Later, two other classmates joined us. Having four people going over the same material left very little chance that we would skip over anything important. Selective study was vital. We could not then, and never would, know it all.

Not everyone was able to keep up. Frederick would be the first classmate to fail out. To be fair, Frederick was never destined to be a physician; that much was clear soon after meeting him. By passion, Frederick was an historian, and by disposition and intellect, he was already an historian of the first order. Much of the history I know, he taught me at lunch or on walks back and forth to the Phi Chi house. Unfortunately, since most of the males in his family had been physicians, he was expected to become a doctor.

We were into the third week of histology, learning to identify the various tissues of the body under the microscope. We usually spent a week on each major tissue, and then had a check-off using all fifty-two microscopes, followed by a four-hour written test.

We had been studying bone, which is one of the more complex and difficult tissues to understand. In addition to knowing about its microscopic appearance and anatomy, we had to know the embryology and how the tissue formed in the fetus. On the day of the exam, Frederick came running up to a small group of us who were waiting in the hallway to go into the lab for the test.

"Hank, for goodness sake, tell me what you know about muscle." Frederick had become so displaced that he had been studying muscle while the rest of us were on bone. The class had finished muscle two weeks ago. Even as he stood there, panicked and flushed, Frederick did not yet realize that he was headed out of medical school.

"MUSCLE?!" Hank yelled. "MUSCLE?! Fred, we are studying bone."

Frederick slumped against the wall and then slid down a few inches. All color drained from his face. "I've been up all night studying muscle. Quick, quick, tell me what you know about bone . . . something. Hell, anything." Hank actually stood there with him and tried to tell him some of the essentials, but it was far too late. Frederick was asked to withdraw after the test, and I never saw him again.

Just after Frederick left, neuroanatomy was added to our workload. Whatever hours had been left to us were gone. Somehow, time had to be made for yet another exhaustive, demanding course. We were forced to steal time from anatomy and histology. Our submersion into medical school was now total. Distant, though important, events like the Korean War vanished from our awareness. There was simply no time for input beyond textbook, laboratory, and lecture notes. Even the immediately discernible aspects of daily life no longer left any impression. One day it was fall; the next day it was the dead of winter. Colors had changed, leaves and then snow had fallen. No time machine could be more effective. We subsisted outside of natural cycles and world events. Only gross anatomy, histology, and neuroanatomy existed.

Neuroanatomy is the study of the structure and function of the brain, the spinal cord, and the peripheral nerves. In order to see the tracts and pathways, the brain was sectioned every few millimeters. The brain and the tracts and nuclei were stained with special stains so they could be identified and seen. Each cross-section was then embedded between two pieces of glass. The trick in learning neuroanatomy was to develop the knack of seeing structures in three dimensions from a two-dimensional section. Nowadays there are all sorts of computer simulations that allow one to display this three-dimensional picture. We had to construct the pictures in our minds.

At night, our group learned to make drawings of the cross-sections at any level of the spinal cord or brain. Hank, being ambidextrous and headed for surgery, would take a piece of chalk in each hand, and with a grand sweep downward of both hands, make the outline of the spinal cord, simultaneously tracing its left and right borders. He repeated this process until he had filled the blackboard with the circular outlines. Then we filled in the various tracts, going higher and higher in the cord until we came to the great crossover zone where everything coming up from the right crosses to the left and vice versa. There was also the great crossover of the descending motor efferent tracts. This crossover of the tracts explains why left-sided strokes produce right-sided deficits and vice versa.

As we progressed in the course, one of us would stand at the blackboard and draw the levels of the cord or brain as the others would make up more and more complex strokes or injuries. "Where would the lesion be that caused paralysis of the right foot and loss of vibration below the right knee but loss of pain, touch, and heat sensation on the left foot?" As we got better and better, we would throw in findings that could only be explained by multiple lesions, such as occur in multiple sclerosis. We played games, taking turns at describing the location of an imaginary destructive lesion. Then the others had to describe the resulting clinical findings that would be produced. This give-and-take and challenge to each other night after night melded the whole of neuroanatomy into one hologram in my mind's eye. To this day, I can follow most of the major tracts up and down the cord and up into the brain, and I can trace the spread as the great tracts sweep their way out onto the cortex—that still amazing symmetry of creation that makes us the highest form of intelligence on the planet, maybe even the universe.

But neuroanatomy represented more than just fascinating study. The immense, near-absurd workload that resulted from its addition forced us to master the fine art of priority juggling. We would work on one subject one day, get one day behind in the other two courses, then catch up in those two and backslide in the third. Again the group study helped. We planned the evening carefully each night, setting time limits to study each course and then moving on, no matter what. This crash course in setting priorities was as vital to our prospects of success as were the medical classes. In the practice of medicine, there is never enough time in one day to get everything done. A doctor never goes to bed with the day's work completely done. We would forever have to decide what was essential, what could wait, and what simply would not get done.

This phantom fourth course, let's call it Priority Juggling 101, would claim the second classmate of the semester. Stockman simply could not distinguish trivial knowledge from important knowledge. Most of us used *Gray's Anatomy* as our text. It had enough detail, but not too much. Stockman used the *Morris Anatomy*. It gave every possible variation and a detailed description of every part of the body.

Though such detailed written descriptions were unnecessary in a visual field, Stockman memorized each and every one. Stockman was a phenomenon. He had an uncanny ability to memorize the written word. At lunch or in the student lounge, we would put him on display to the upper class students. We would say, "Stockman, tell them what the kidney looks like."

He would stand, look off into the distance, and begin. "The kidney, also known as the renal organ, lies in a posterior position in the retro-peritoneal space. Its outer, lateral border is convex, while its medial border is concave where the renal pelvis forms a saccular body draining caudally into the ureter. The left kidney, on it cephalad tip, lies under the tail of the pancreas and a portion of the splenic flexure of the transverse colon . . ." On and on he would go, reciting the exact words from Morris's textbook. We would follow him in the book as he recited, and marvel as he left no conjunction out or adjective misplaced. He did this for all the parts of the body, and especially the shapes of all the bones and the sites of attachments of the ligaments and muscles. This was a *tour de force* of memory, but he missed the big picture. He could not find the parts in the cadaver, and spent little time dissecting. For Stockman, anatomy was a verbal exercise rather than a visual one. He failed every check-off where he tried to recite his memorized descriptions. Anatomy demanded hands-on knowledge, not textbook passages. By the end of the first semester, Stockman was asked to with-draw. Unlike Frederick, his departure caught me by surprise. I had thought he had only memorized the descriptions to get laughs, which he invariably did. No one seriously thought he believed that the ability to deliver *Morris Anatomy*–informed monologues was what anatomy was all about. He must have been more surprised than any of us.

Frederick and Stockman illustrated a simple truth of med school. Most medical students who fail out do not fail for lack of brainpower. They fail because they either give up or they are lazy or they are unmo-tivated. They fail because partial attention will not suffice. During my years of study, students failed because they were sloppy, because they could not set priorities, because their concentration lapsed for a month or a week or even a day. But no student failed for lack of mental power. They failed because the raw desire has to be intense to survive this first year of medical school. And unlike intellect, desire is not measured in wattage. Desire is measured by the weight it can bear and by the pressure it can withstand.

Gross anatomy, histology, neuroanatomy, and even Priority Juggling 101 were all just components of a single, simple, vital test of desire. By the semester's end, all but two of us could look in the mirror and see a person who, though weary, dateless, and remarkably uninformed about world events, had borne the weight and withstood the pressure. More tests lay ahead, and more failures were certain, but for a moment we were triumphant.

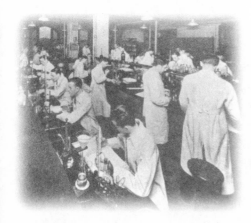

3

QUAIL
HUNTING

The building of the School of Medicine and Hospital is located in the south east corner of the University Campus. It is constructed in the collegiate Gothic style, the structure being of concrete with brick and limestone walls . . . the building is in reality a series of buildings brought together so that they are all under one roof . . . The entire plant is so arranged that there is free communication between the various departments of the School and Hospital, and the library, with its spacious reading room in the center of the building. The Medical School is so arranged to accommodate two hundred students.

The Outpatient Service occupies the entire first floor of the southern portion of the building. It is especially designed for teaching and contains a series of examining, treatment, and teaching rooms for general medicine and surgery, pediatrics, neurology, dermatology, psychiatry, dentistry, orthopedic surgery, ophthalmology, otolaryngology, obstetrics, gynecology, and urology . . . A waiting room adjoins each department and several small clinical laboratories are placed in convenient locations.

Catalogue for 1951–1952
School of Medicine
Vanderbilt University

THREE TIGHTLY CONNECTED BUILDINGS FORMED THE medical school/hospital complex. On the north end, there were the faculty offices and the teaching laboratories of the basic science departments. On the south end were the inpatient wards and the outpatient clinics. The middle building contained the offices of the clinical faculty.

15

On any floor we could walk from a laboratory in basic science to a clinician's office to the hospital ward or clinic. The theory behind the layout was that clinical problems at the bedside could be taken directly to the research laboratories of the basic scientists. The physical intimacy put science and clinical medicine side by side. It was a perfectly designed medical school.

During our study group's breaks, Hank sometimes led us on reconnaissance missions. Some nights he went alone. By mid-October, Hank had explored the entire hospital/medical school complex. He knew every turn and corner of the complicated maze. One night on our late night break, Hank came running into the cafeteria. He was giggling and talking at the same time, a distracting habit he had when he was excited. It made him totally unintelligible until he stopped laughing. Finally he said, "Come on. Now. You've got to see this one."

It was not unusual for Hank to return from reconnoitering and drag us off to one discovery or another. One night he found the autopsy room. We sneaked in and got the pathology resident to show us the fresh anatomy of an autopsy. It was the first time I had seen the insides of a body that had not been completely embalmed and cured in formalin. There was little similarity between the fresh tissues of the autopsy and the dried flesh of our cadaver. The cadaver seemed an abstraction of the real body, so far removed from death that we no longer thought of it as coming from a real person. At the autopsy, on the other hand, organs glistened and reflected light. The heart was purple, not a pale, dried-out brown. The lungs were pink and stood up, still filled with air from the last breath of the dying patient.

On another night Hank found the delivery room, and we watched a baby being born. Within a week, Hank's scouting expeditions had leapt from the end of life to its beginnings. I will never forget the wonder of seeing a new human coming into life. At first the baby was motionless, all wet and reddish blue. Blood was everywhere. For an instant I thought the baby was stillborn. Suddenly, the lifeless form erupted and gave forth one long wail after another. Each cry forced the lungs further open to receive air. I thought it strange that birth and death, the first and last human acts, are bathed in crying and tears. Crying is essential for life.

On this particular night, Hank was unusually excited. We loped off after him as he half-walked, half-ran out of the cafeteria. We could hear him giggling as he turned one corner after another in the maze of hallways. Soon we were in a darkened section of the first floor headed toward the clinics. We could barely make out his outline in the dim light.

"Shh . . . Be quiet. No talking." Hank held up his hand to halt the three of us following him. We were marines sneaking up on some unknown enemy position. "Pretty soon now . . . now . . . now watch this." Hank whispered, still giggling under his breath at the same time.

With that, he yanked a large lever on the wall of the clinic, and the entire long corridor and all rooms off to the sides burst into light. He had found the master electrical switch for a whole wing. Every space in the long clinic lit up. We stood there surprised at the sudden brilliance that replaced the dark.

Hank whispered, "Hold, hold."

At the far end of the long corridor, first one, then two, finally a third janitor came out of the rooms, each sweeping as furiously as possible. Hank motioned for us to walk toward the three men.

"Good evening," Hank said, suppressing his giggles and rushing off into one of the clinic teaching conference rooms. We collapsed into the chairs, covered our mouths, and forced ourselves not to laugh out loud.

The men had obviously been loafing on the job, and from their appearance, it was obvious they had been asleep in the clinic exam rooms. Wakened by the lights, they feigned activity and came out sweeping, as if—moments before in the pitch black—they had been sweeping just as vigorously.

Hank dubbed it "janitor quail hunting." For those of us raised in rural areas, it was an apt name. He spoke of cover shots, of hunting down the singles, and of getting one, two, even three shots on the covey rise. Hank honed janitor quail hunting to an art.

At first we hunted every night, and soon enough there were no janitors anywhere. Hank said we had overhunted the fields. So we started waiting about a week between hunts. Sure enough, the janitor population recovered and stabilized, and we could count on one or two, and—on good nights—three janitors in each clinic, always coming out sweeping when the lights went on.

Hank had made certain migratory discoveries about where the janitors next alighted. He had found that the general medical clinic janitors tended to fly to the GYN clinic, while the surgical clinic janitors regularly drifted to the pediatric clinic.

There was one stretch of several weeks where we flushed no coveys. We stopped hunting for two weeks, but there were still no janitors. We were puzzled by the disappearances. Hank assured us they were out there somewhere. We just had to find them.

After more than a month of no success, Hank rushed into the cafeteria. "Those damn sophomores. I caught them poaching janitors up in the orthopedic clinic. No wonder our hunting dried up. You can't overshoot a field and expect to find birds. Those guys don't know a damn thing about quail hunting or game conservation."

At times there were no bounds on our need for humor.

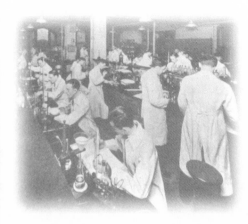

4

BEWARE
OF
DEAD DOGS

521. Physiology. — This course for first-year medical students is designed to cover the essentials of medical physiology. Twenty hours per week of lectures, conferences, and laboratory work are given during the second semester of the first year.

Catalogue for 1951–1952
School of Medicine
Vanderbilt University

THE SECOND SEMESTER OF THE FIRST YEAR STARTED heavy: biochemistry with two labs a week, physiology with two labs, another two months of neuroanatomy, an introduction to pharmacology, and a course in biostatistics.

The physiology department consisted of three faculty members. We dubbed this trinity "Aged P.," "Madman," and "Chinaman." Dr. King was "Aged P." The nickname stood for aged professor, a take-off on Dickens's "aged parent." Dr. King was in his late seventies and had been brought back out of retirement. Like some ancient priest with a benevolent face, he made his daily tour of the laboratory, nodding here and there as he passed our tables in the laboratory. I would not have been too surprised if he had swung a pot of incense to bless our work.

The "Madman" was Dr. Robert Post, a young instructor who had just finished his post-doctoral at Harvard. Post rode a Harley-Davidson to work, occasionally came to class wearing Lederhosen and a feathered Alpine cap, and came by his eccentricity honestly—he was a genius.

The "Chinaman," the third and most junior of the trinity, was a Chinese physiologist who had arrived in the country a few years before. Dr. Ray Meng had already made some fundamental observations on parenteral nutrition, and would later make intravenous fat available for patients with absent gut function. Later in his career, he would gain national renown for his extensive studies in nutrition. But in Vanderbilt's physiology department in 1951, our class knew only one thing about Dr. Meng: we could understand very little of what he said.

Twice a week we had afternoon labs. As the junior faculty member, Dr. Meng's main duty was to supervise the afternoon laboratory sessions. These sessions called for complicated preparations. We started with frogs, pigeons, and small fish, then squids and rats. Each experiment required extensive prep time to get the equipment all set up and the primitive recording devices ready to measure whatever it was the experiment required. Toward the end of the course we moved to dogs.

The work group consisted of four students. We kept our same cadaver group, which was a testament to how well we got along. Given the tensions and near fights over the head and neck dissection, many cadaver groups split up. Jean, Oscar, Hank, and I would work at one table. For each experiment in physiology we assigned roles. One of us would be head surgeon, one anesthesiologist, one engineer, and one scut boy. By far the worst role was that of scut boy. We rotated the roles so that none of us got stuck as scut boy more than any other. Scut boy had to get the smoked drum set up and done.

We did not have the advanced electronic recording devices that are commonplace in any laboratory today; they had not yet been invented. We used rotating metal drums, around which we wrapped a thick piece of paper that was then coated with thick black smoke. The paper was first attached around the entire drum. Then the drum was slowly rotated in a kerosene flame device, allowing the smoke to coat the drum evenly. This sounds simple, but it was tedious, and it took a lot of practice to coat the drum just right. Too little smoke and the quill writer would not leave a tracing. Too much smoke and the writer would smudge or, worse, the entire layer of smoke would just peel off the paper. The smoked drum was then placed near the animal and a sharpened goose quill was attached to the lever device. The lever was then attached to a muscle or duct or whatever was going to cause a motion or flow that could be measured. The goose quill scratched the surface of the slowly turning drum and left a tracing of the motion. In addition to this motion quill, we had a timer quill, sometimes an EKG quill, and on big experiments, additional motion quills. Occasionally, we accidentally smudged the smoke and had to start all over—from the beginning of the experiment. With luck, we could get the dog anesthetized, the dissection done, the drum smoked, have all the devices attached, and be ready for the experiment in two to three hours. But there was a big catch.

If the dog died before three hours, the group had to start over from the beginning. If the dog died after three hours, we could stop the experiment wherever we were, calculate the results, make the record permanent by spraying the drum with shellac, clean up, and go home by 6:00 P.M. If the dog died too early, we had to start the experiment over. This meant finishing sometimes as late as 9:00 or 10:00 P.M.

The two tables next to ours were studies in contrast. To our right, the students were singularly technically inept. Nothing ever went right. They rarely ever got the drum smoked correctly. The dog was usually either wide awake or so deep in anesthesia they had to bag-breathe it to keep it alive. None of the preparation was done correctly. The little ducts we were to cannulate were torn beyond use. And then to cap it all off, their dog would die at exactly three hours and five minutes, letting them off the hook. According to the three-hour rule, they could calculate their results from whatever they had collected and legally borrow data from adjoining tables to finish the work. This meant they were through by 4:00 P.M. and could leave. Despite their ability to get out of work, they complained the entire time and detested all laboratory work. None wanted to be the surgeon or do any part of the experimental work. Each wanted to keep the notes, or make the observations, but stay away from any mechanical tasks. They were all mind and no hands. We could tell then that they had psychiatric career tendencies.

The group to our left was the polar opposite in mechanical competence from the table of future psychiatrists. Even at that early date, one could tell that this group was destined to become surgeons. The group constantly argued about their roles. There was shoving and loud talk about who would make incisions, who would do the detailed dissections, or who would get to do the most of the scut preparations. They actually *fought* over who would get to do the scut work. Roles were usually assigned by coin flip, and even then they complained constantly. Despite the arguments, they were extremely hard-working and diligent with the experiments, invariably producing the best and cleanest experimental results. They even took pride in how the results were presented. The rest of us cared, but our major objective was to get done and learn the point of the experiment. For this group, the doing of the experiment was the main thing.

One afternoon we heard raised voices from the surgeon group to our left. There was arguing and shoving in their usual fashion, and then things became real quiet. Then we heard a lot of whispering. Suddenly, one of the group declared in a loud voice, "Damn, our dog has died." It was an exaggerated and rehearsed announcement, and it reminded me of a self-conscious fourth grader in a grammar-school play. The careful diction and loud voice betrayed what had really happened.

Whenever a dog died after the magical three-hour limit, Dr. Meng had to inspect the situation and make a ruling on the death. With deaths too soon after the three-hour limit, there was always a nagging suspicion that the students had let the dog die in order to finish sooner.

Meng approached the table. He walked around one side then another. He looked at the color of the dog's tongue, our ever-available window to oxygenation. The tongue showed the blue black sign of death.

Hank loved to imitate Meng's response. In the lounge Hank would look one way, then turn his head and look another way, then make like he was looking under the table. Then he would put his hands on his hips and say, in a loud poorly imitated Chinese accent, "Dog dead."

Pause. "Dog not die. Boys kill dog. Must do experiment over."

Dr. Meng did not let anything get by him.

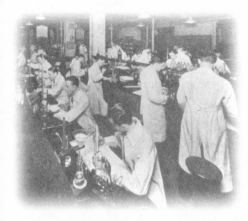

5

MYASTHENIA GRAVIS

5. Special Clinical Lectures and Demonstrations. — A series of clinical lectures and demonstration for the purpose of bringing before the class patients illustrating unusual and important diseases.

Catalogue for 1951–1952
School of Medicine
Vanderbilt University

IN THE FIRST YEAR AND A HALF OF MEDICAL SCHOOL, ALL the focus is on science. So naturally, as the courses went by, we became more and more interested in seeing live patients. I remember our first exposure to a real patient. We were in the middle of the nervous system in physiology in the last part of the first year, waiting for the lecturer to appear, when the doors of the amphitheater opened. An attendant rolled a wheelchair into the bottom of the theater. A white-haired woman who appeared to be in her fifties sat slumped to one side in the wheelchair. She was the most pitiful person I had ever seen. Her mouth was half open with drool dripping down from one corner. She struggled to raise her head from its dangling position, but could not. Her eyes were half closed. It was obvious that the woman was paralyzed.

We were then introduced to Dr. Sam Riven, her physician and a member of the clinical faculty. Dr. Riven told us the woman had myasthenia gravis. We had been studying the neuromuscular junction and its associated neurotransmitters. The acetylcholine and cholinesterase reactions were familiar to us, so we were prepared to understand some of what we saw and heard.

Dr. Riven told us that the patient had agreed to omit one dose of her medicines so we could see how she appeared untreated. The woman made a feeble effort to smile with ever so slight movement of the corners of her mouth, and a hoarse whispery sound when she tried to laugh. He then asked her to perform several tasks. He held up an arm and then let go. The arm flopped back into her lap. She could not move her legs or arms, could not raise her head, could not open her eyes. She could swallow, but could not speak, at least in a voice we could hear. Dr. Riven kept patting her on the head and reassuring her. He asked her if she could tolerate a few more minutes. She made a barely noticeable nod of her head. It was more like she raised her head a fraction of an inch and then let go as her head bobbled a few times on her chest.

Dr. Riven then took a filled syringe from his black bag. He held the syringe high in the air and squirted a small spray from the needle, swabbed the patient's upper arm, and injected the clear liquid into the patient. We sat there in complete silence for a few minutes. Slowly the woman came alive. At first she was able to fully open her eyes, then she could close her mouth, then she raised her head to an upright position. The drooling stopped. Very slowly she adjusted her position in the wheelchair. And then, like a pure miracle, she sat upright, stood up, spread her arms out to each side, and made a small bow as if to say, "Here I am." We applauded and began talking to each other.

She went on to tell us in a clear and strong voice how Dr. Riven had made the diagnosis a year ago, and how her life had been brought back nearly to normal by his treatment with physostigmine. Early in the course of her disease, several doctors had missed the diagnosis. They told her she was just neurotic. She would be forever grateful to Dr. Riven, and was glad to be able to show us medical students what the disease was like. Maybe that would keep us from missing the diagnosis as had happened in her case.

It amazed me then, and it still amazes me, that science had identified the details of neuromuscular transmission, isolated and named its chemical compounds, identified the biochemical lesion in mysasthenia gravis, and then synthesized a drug to counteract the chemical defect that produced the disease.

The fifty years that have passed since this demonstration have in no way lessened its impact on me. The moment Dr. Riven's patient stood up, I knew that I wanted to be able to have that effect on a patient, to be able to make diagnoses, to treat patients, and to give a normal life back to those who have been afflicted. I naively thought all diseases would be like myasthenia gravis. I pictured medicine as finding some missing chemical or element, then supplying the missing substance, and curing the patient. I somehow thought all diseases and their remedies would be as straightforward as what we had just witnessed. I believed medical science would find similar cures for every single disease, and that I would live long enough to make all kinds of diagnoses, give a pill or an injection, and cure people completely. At that time I saw medicine as limitless. What was not curable then was only what had not been worked out through science.

I have practiced and taught medicine for almost fifty years. I have not made a diagnosis of myasthenia gravis in a single patient, although I have looked for the disease diligently. Although several people with the disease have been in my practice, I have never made the original diagnosis. It took many years for me to see that not only was myasthenia gravis a very rare disease, but that there would be few other diseases as clearly defined or as dramatically treatable, at least in my lifetime.

And you know, maybe I am still naive, but I believe that woman who came to life after an injection in 1952 epitomizes the effect that medicine and the scientific method will eventually have on all diseases. I remain in complete awe of the power of the scientific method. It may be humanity's single greatest achievement.

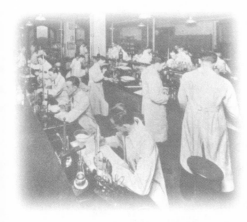

6

THE FIRST
HOUSE CALL

No grades regarding their relative scholastic standing are given to students.
Students who fail in two major courses at any time during their medical course
year or fail a re-examination in a major course may be required to withdraw from
the school. Students who have had no reported failures may be required to with-
draw from the school if their work has been of a generally unsatisfactory quality.

Students will be notified whenever the Committee on Promotions considers their
work of poor quality, thus serving notice of the necessity for greater effort in order
to carry the work of the school.

Catalogue for 1951–1952
School of Medicine
Vanderbilt University

DEAN JOHN YOUMANS INTRODUCED A NEW COURSE IN
the fall of the first semester of our first year. It was not listed in the
catalogue, but just appeared. We were in the middle of gross anatomy,
histology, and just beginning neuroanatomy when the dean decided
we should be introduced, "as early as possible to family dynamics."
Each of us was assigned a family to follow for all four years of medical
school. We were to make two home visits each semester to see our
families. Although the basic idea of humanizing medicine was sound
and far ahead of most medical schools at that time, the timing could
not have been worse.

"Social and Environmental Medicine," as the dean called it, began just after Thanksgiving. Once a week we spent two hours of desperately needed study time with one of the four psychiatric social workers assigned to each group of thirteen medical students. Families were presented and discussed by the social worker. During this period, Freudian psychiatry was at its zenith across academic America. There was no other school of psychological thought admitted. None. No Carl Jung, no Carl Rogers, no Alfred Adler, or any of the other extant theorists of that time. Freud was king of psychiatry, an absolute monarch, not to be questioned. Every behavior at every stage of development was traced by our group's social worker to sexual jealousy or inhibitions or repression. Whatever lasting value Freud's theories may have had on the rest of the world was lost on most of our class through the dogmatic presentations of the social workers. At least that is the way we were taught it, or maybe that was the way some of us took it in.

The social worker leading our group stressed that early toilet training reigned king of all formative forces. Everything in the conferences was referenced either to anal-retentive behavior from overly strict toilet training, or to loosely organized social structure from overly loose toilet training. The Oedipal complex was mentioned with every family history. Favorite phrases were "penis envy" for misbehaving little girls, fear of "oral conception" for any feeding problem in a young girl, and lust for either parent, albeit submerged and repressed. The subconscious was a dark and unfriendly place, with neuroses lurking, waiting to surface at some later time in some unknown place.

If anyone challenged any of the Freudian concepts, the standard answer from the social worker was, "I can see that you are obviously threatened by that idea. Is there something you want to tell us?" It was a stopper of the first order. First of all, we were at the height of testosterone production, locked up in a gross anatomy lab, and unable to get a date because of the stench of formalin. We were, thus, highly unlikely to share repressed sexual fantasies with the female social workers. It didn't happen. Perhaps the real fear was that if we started talking, we would just reveal everything, and some hideous repression would come bubbling out, beyond our control to stop. All of this was going on long before the birth control pill or the so-called sexual revolution. Sex and any discussion of it were just emerging from the Victorian age, which had denied its existence in any civilized conversation.

The course work assumed that we were to take all of this Freudian terminology in and use it on our home visit interviews. Following these interviews, we were to do detailed write-ups of our visits. By January no one in my group had made the first home visit. We were, almost as a class, in complete passive-aggressive rebellion. Most of my classmates felt the same way I did. We simply did not have the time or inclination to ride a bus halfway across town, visit a family we had never met, interview them using tools we did not understand, and then do a lengthy write-up on a subject we did not comprehend.

The longer we failed to visit, the angrier the dean became. His anger peaked in late January just before the semester ended. We were called to a special meeting of the class. It was our first meeting with the dean since the first day of school.

Dean John Youmans came hobbling in on crutches, his right leg in a thigh-length cast. We knew he had fallen off his horse on one of his hound hunts and fractured his lower leg. The dean liked bourbon. He liked fox hunting. He liked horses. He liked to jump them. Word was that he got into the bourbon a little early on his last hunt.

This day he was furious. We could tell by the set of his small mouth when he came in the door. Small already, his mouth was pursed into a tiny pencil-size hole. We soon learned to judge his anger by the size of his mouth. His face was red, and his hair, usually plastered down tight, was slightly uncombed. The "Four Freudian Bitches," our group's name for the four social workers, filed into the steep amphitheater. They looked equally unhappy about our failure to comply.

The dean hobbled to the podium in the pit of the amphitheater. "This class has been a problem from the very beginning. First of all, you did not know it, but you are the first class ever to be interviewed as part of the selection process. My faculty told me I was making a mistake to do that, and I now agree. They have joked with me and chided me and called you quote 'the personality whiz class' unquote. Well their fears were well founded."

He continued that ours would be the last class interviewed, and that we were a disgrace to the school. That our refusal to do what was required in a course was not acceptable, and that unless each of us had a written report of at least one home visit on his desk by the end of January, he would fail the entire class if he needed to. He stipulated that there was no requirement to have a class of '55, and that he and the school could just skip a year of graduation without missing it. He was far beyond fed up; he was at his wit's end. When he finished, he hobbled out of the door, with the psychiatric social workers following behind him.

As we slumped out of the amphitheater, I began to lay plans for the dreaded home visit to see my family. We knew the dean was serious and that he would follow through on failing us. He was known as a man of his word, and he had not wasted any in his short talk. Out of pure fear, we would make the house calls and write the reports.

My assigned family lived on the opposite side of town from the medical school. It would take a long bus ride downtown and then two transfers to get there. Other than the town students, only the married veterans and a couple of others owned cars. The rest of us were on foot. Ordinarily, I would have bummed a ride from Hank, but this time everyone was so frantic to make the home visit, we were all scurrying on our own. We only had five days to make the visits and write the reports. I set aside an afternoon for the visit. One of the social workers had scheduled it for me.

The families had been selected through the Obstetrics clinic; thus, the women in these families were pregnant and would deliver sometime in the next several months. One idea behind the program was for us to follow a woman through labor and delivery, to see the impact of a new baby on family dynamics, and to see the child through early childhood. At one level we knew the course had some merit, but at another level we knew an F in Social and Environmental

Medicine would not be as bad as an F in anatomy, histology, or neuroanatomy. This assumption, coupled with the condescending attitude of the social workers, put the kiss of death on any hopes for the program's success. They did not like our class, and most of us did not like them.

The first leg of my bus ride left me downtown. I was beginning to feel a little queasy, given my lifelong disposition to motion sickness. If back seat car rides produced nausea, imagine what a bus ride— complete with fumes—did for me. By the end of the first transfer, I was well into terminal nausea. I let one bus go by while I sat on the curb, trying not to vomit, knowing I could not possibly make the full ride of the final transfer without losing my lunch. I held on for the last leg of the trip until I got to my final stop. Then my mouth filled with hot saliva. I was soaking wet with sweat. Mercifully, I was able to step off the bus as soon as the door opened and barf. I was drenched in sweat, sick as I could get, and I felt like I would faint if I did not lie down. The blast of cold January air was the only thing that helped me to recover.

The bus ride landed me in a poor section of town. The streets were in need of paving, and the shoulders of the roads ran off into washed-out ruts. The small gullies ended at the ditches along the roads. There were two cars jacked up on concrete blocks standing in a patch of high brown weeds on the vacant corner lot. An old rusting school bus with all of the windows broken out was sitting on its axles at the back of the vacant lot. I crawled into the bus and noted my sorry appearance in the cracked mirror. My hair was soaking wet with perspiration. My color was pale gray, with my lips blending into my face. I lay on the front seat of the bus exhausted, sweaty, and still nauseated. Thankfully, motion sickness passes once the motion stops, and after a few minutes I recovered. The cold air finished its job, and in less than half an hour, I had dried off, put back on my coat and tie, and was up and heading toward my family's house a few blocks away.

A moment after my knock on the door, a little girl, maybe seven years old, answered it. When she opened it, a wave of hot air rushed by me. The temperature inside must have been more than eighty degrees. The mother quickly appeared by her daughter's side. Both were sweating from the heat, and both looked tired. The mother was pregnant. The smells of wet laundry, ironing, and gas heat filled the air.

"You must be one of them Vanderbilt doctors," she said, drying her hands on her apron. "The social worker told me you was coming. Come on in."

The house was quite small, but very neat. I wondered if the mother had some disease that required high heat, but I did not follow up on the idea. The mother took the chair across from me, and her little girl hid behind the chair. The living room also served as the dining room. There was a sofa, two chairs, and a round table in one corner. The walls were bare painted wood. The only picture was a photograph of a man in a World War II Army uniform. It hung over the mantle.

I smiled and thanked them for having me in. Then the room went silent. I could not think of anything to say. Now that I look back on it, there was some sort of cultural chasm I could not bridge. The woman said nothing. The little girl said nothing. I said nothing. We sat and looked at each other. I could hear a kettle somewhere in the back of the house making a fine-pitched hissing. I could hear the clock on the mantle ticking. My anxiety finally got to me. I said something inane like, "I guess you visit the clinic."

The mother said, "Yes." Nothing more. No expansion on the idea. Trying to talk with her was like talking into a wind. Nothing came back. Every time I thought of something to ask, all I got was a monosyllabic response and then silence except for the sounds of the house. I could even hear the open gas heater in front of the fireplace making a faint hum and hiss.

I was becoming more anxious. I was groping by now and a very long way from getting up the nerve to ask about toilet training or weaning from the breast, subjects we had been told to explore. Somehow I had to broach the subjects. "Your daughter looks healthy," I said. Somehow I thought that opening could lead me to get up the nerve to ask about toilet training. It didn't.

"Well, she ain't." The mother said, still staring at me.

"Oh, what's the matter?" I asked, sensing another opening.

"You ain't a real doctor is you?" the mother said. And then a long pause. "Nancy's got the asthma. Least ways, she had the asthma real bad 'til we bought her Twitty."

At that point, Nancy came around the edge of the chair and held out a purse toward me. "Show him Twitty, Nancy. Show him," the mother said, pushing Nancy toward me.

I looked into the open purse, and there sat a bedraggled parakeet, looking up at me and jerking its head from side to side. He made no effort to escape. The bird looked like he had just come out of a bath, feathers all wet and stuck together. Nancy then told me about her pet bird, how she bathed it every day in the kitchen sink. Since she got the bird, her asthma had gone away. At least that's what the mother insisted.

I didn't know anything about asthma and nothing about birds curing asthma or anything about anything they had brought up. I felt stupid and out of place. All I wanted to do was leave, get out of there. Every pretense at intelligent conversation failed. Every question they asked, I couldn't honestly answer. Every question I asked evoked only one-word responses. I was useless. Worse, the mother knew I was useless. Would she tell the social workers, and would they run and tell the dean, and would he call me in and fail me out of medical school? What would I put in my written report?

After a few more minutes of silence and short responses, I said I had to be going. The mother said good-bye. Nancy waved from the door as I looked back toward the house. I had accomplished nothing. What was I supposed to have done? I didn't come close to asking about toilet training or weaning from the breast. All I could do was dread the bus ride to the hospital. Somehow I got back without vomiting again. The entire trip took nearly four hours. I was beat.

The write-up I submitted detailed the story of my motion sickness, the wet parakeet, and the miraculous remission of the girl's asthma. I had completely forgotten to ask about the husband and father during my visit. I just assumed the photograph was the husband, so I mentioned a "military background." My highly buffed report did not capture the full truth of the dismal experience. I had gone to the literature for my report, and so I beefed it up considerably. I spent some time on the socio-economic conditions of the neighborhood. I even mentioned my concerns for parrot fever (psittacosis), having found out that the family of birds that included parakeets could transmit a special type of pneumonia. I thought it added a bit of scientific class to the report. The social workers did not, and they belittled me for not attending to the Freudian maxims.

I never saw my assigned family again. We continued to meet with the social workers every two weeks for another month or so. And then, like a miracle, the course vanished. No announcement—it just got canceled. We think the basic science faculty decided it was too intrusive on the "real" science we should have been learning. I learned years later that the course surfaced again in 1955. Well planned and better designed, the course would have been an excellent idea. Dean Youmans and Vanderbilt were far ahead of the times with the idea of humanizing medical education, a topic under much discussion a few years later. The idea of following the developments in one family for four years was sound. Unfortunately, the instruction was exclusively Freudian and ill-timed in the midst of the first semester of the first year. At any rate, our passive aggression won out. Wally, on hearing our stories, said we were all anal retentive.

No one in my group had a good experience on the visit. The only thing good about the whole affair was that it was now behind us.

For the rest of the semester, we went back to full effort on neuroanatomy, histology, and the remaining parts of the head and neck. Hard sciences won out over the soft theories of the psyche.

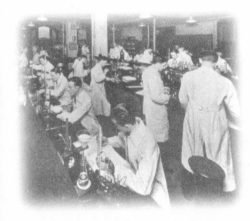

7

STUDIES IN
CONTRAST
AND SEPARATION

Special Elective Courses. — A limited number of students . . . may be accepted for special elective work each trimester in the various laboratories of the departments.
Catalogue for 1951–1952
School of Medicine
Vanderbilt University

I DECIDED TO STAY IN NASHVILLE FOR THE SUMMER AFTER my freshman year. I had an interesting offer to work as a research assistant at the Veterans Administration Hospital doing dog surgery for a cardiology drug study. Hank had worked it out for both of us. Another classmate, John, would also be working with us. I would get paid enough to live on if I stayed in my room at the Phi Chi house. Jean had taken over as house manager and was working as a counselor and bus driver for a children's day camp. Oscar had gone to his farm in Arkansas for the summer. A number of other classmates were also taking summer jobs as elective courses, so I looked forward to the camaraderie in addition to the chance to taste research work up close.

In order to keep the Phi Chi house open for the summer, Jean had negotiated a deal to rent the entire house, except for our rooms, to a group of high school coaches who returned each summer to attend Peabody College. In three summers they would get a master's degree in physical education. As one of them put it, "Hell, I'm away from the old lady all summer. I'll get a raise in pay when I get my master's.

What else could you ask for?" It was going to be a summer of contrasts.

Despite coming from different high schools spread across the southeast, the coaches seemed to know each other very well. Most of them had attended Peabody for a summer or two before, and under the leadership of the "veterans," deployment into their new environs was swift. Within the first day the beachhead was established. They had set up a sizable bar area in the living room and had pulled back all the furniture to make a dance floor. One of the men installed a record player and speakers in the hall, and they even made some half-hearted efforts to clean up the first floor area. By the second day the place looked like a small nightclub. By the third night, anyone wanting to carouse and drink was free to join. The parties began and continued nightly nearly all summer.

Each day Hank picked me up in front of the Phi Chi house in his 1941 Chevy, and we drove to the VA Hospital. The car was on its last few miles, and it took Hank hours each week to keep the thing going. First it was the carburetor, then the muffler, then the radiator, and finally the pistons. Hank related everything to medical practice. He thought of the carburetor as a heart and gasoline as blood. He spoke of major surgery, critical care, being in the recovery room. He would not accept my suggestion that the car was terminal. He said it was only in mild congestive heart failure.

The car looked rough. The cloth lining in the ceiling had been partially ripped out, leaving the sheet metal of the roof exposed. The front seats were blown out from some obese previous owner, so that I sat on a front seat that leaned severely back and to the right. The back seat was missing. Hank used that space to carry two spare tires. (He averaged a flat tire every few weeks.) The car was gassy, constantly sputtering, backfiring, and emitting clouds of black smoke. Having lost its muffler long ago, I could hear Hank coming a block away. And so could the coaches, for whom the decrepit vehicle was a steady source of amusement. They offered to buy it from Hank for five dollars, or to junk it for him if he would pay them.

But whether the car's condition was terminal or mild, a car ride was better than a forty-five-minute bus ride with a transfer. With my experience on the bus during the recent home visit debacle still vivid in my mind, *any* alternative was preferable.

The Thayer VA Hospital was out in the country, on the edge of town about eight miles from downtown. The hospital had been built to receive and treat returning wounded from World War II just a few years before. At its peak, the census could be expanded to more than two thousand beds. Thousands of returning military personnel had been treated at the hospital until its use as a military hospital ended in 1946, at which time it was converted into the Veterans Hospital.

The huge complex sat in the middle of a large pastoral area with nothing close by except a public golf course that abutted one edge of the property. Along another side of the campus were rows of wooden barracks, where some of the married veteran medical students and house officers could get low-cost housing. For me these barracks served an additional function. They reaffirmed my decision to remain single, at least through medical school. One good look at those barracks did it. They looked like the back end of a slum. Laundry was stretched from one unit to another. A few scattered bikes lay here and there. In between two of the barracks, someone had pulled together a few lawn chairs and a table with a torn umbrella tilted against it. It was a depressing sight.

Down the street at one corner of the large property was an open air movie theater for the veterans. An outdoor swimming pool for the patients and their families was between the theater and the married student barracks at the front of the sprawling campus. It was a non-exclusive country club on a tight budget.

The hospital itself consisted of five half-mile long corridors connected by closed passageways. Down the long corridors were attached wooden barracks every fifty yards or so. Each barrack served as a ward that could house up to forty patients. It was designed like the original Army post hospitals from the 1800s, on the theory that if an epidemic broke out in one barrack, you could simply burn it down and contain the contagion. Also, if fire broke out, you would lose only one unit and quickly control the fire from spreading.

It took us about fifteen minutes to walk from the dog lab at one corner of the hospital to the mess hall on the opposite corner. It was a trip we took each day at noon. The free lunch was another perk which made the summer job all the more attractive. Hank and I were constantly low on money. Most of the time we were completely out of any cash. Free food was a big attraction at any time.

Each day we walked the long corridors that undulated and followed the gentle rise and fall of the land. We could barely see the end of the halls as they faded into small points in the distance. All along the way, opposite each ward, double doors opened directly to the outside. The veterans hovered around each doorway. They sat, stood, or squatted in small groups, talking in low tones and smoking. Cigarettes were ten cents a pack, and the canteen carried all brands. In addition, the women volunteers brought cigarettes around to the wards along with magazines and candy. Smoking was nearly universal among the veterans. The association of smoking with lung disease had not yet been established.

All the patients wore wrinkled denim uniforms consisting of white T-shirts, dark green open-front jackets, and pajama-looking pants with a tie cord. They reminded me of pictures of Japanese prisoners of war, who always seemed to be in pajamas in their photographs.

The census of the hospital was around eight hundred at any one time. Most of the patients were on full ambulatory status, waiting for some test result, to recover fully from some procedure, or to have elective surgery. Length of stay was of no concern for anyone—patients or doctors. Those who were waiting for tests often had to wait for a week or two to get the ordered X-rays or special procedures. They sat around, went to the canteen, or ambled out to the swimming pool. The complex, with its slow-moving population all dressed exactly alike, was like a large minimum security prison, with everyone on the honor system.

Each day in the lab, Hank, John, and I prepared for the experiments of the day. Since there were three of us doing the animal experiments, one of us acted as anesthesiologist, one as surgeon, and the third as scrub nurse. The procedure required an infusion of one of several drugs followed by the induction of ventricular fibrillation by occluding the left coronary artery for thirty minutes and then releasing the occlusion. A predictable number of dogs would fibrillate under those conditions. We were testing to see which drugs and what doses would prevent the fibrillation. It was fascinating work, and we learned about experimental design, the difficulties with repetitive experiments, and the statistical analysis that went along with that method of drug testing.

Dr. George Meneely ran the research laboratory. In addition to our research, there were other groups working on an artificial heart and lung machine, another measuring the effects of high sodium diets in rats, and others attempting to define the vitamin requirements of humans. It was quite a varied group, and it reflected Meneely's far-reaching interests.

To say Dr. Meneely was a large man doesn't put it quite right. He was huge, massive, gargantuan. At six feet three inches he was tall, but on top of that he weighed more than 350 pounds. Some large men wear their trousers under the belly bulge, and some wear them over the bulge, but Meneely wore his directly on the greatest diameter of his considerable belly. His waist must have been in excess of sixty inches.

Three afternoons a week, Dr. Meneely directed Hank, John, and me to hear him lecture in the auditorium down the hall from the lab. The scene had a surrealistic character to it. The auditorium could seat more than three hundred people, yet there were only the three of us. The first day we thought we were just early for Meneely's talk. We soon found out that we were the only audience, and would be for the rest of the summer. Why he chose to lecture in the large, hot auditorium instead of his conference room is still a puzzle. The stage was equipped for a full theatrical presentation, with heavy stage curtains, lighting, and all of the paraphernalia of a theater.

The whole thing was quite formal. We sat there waiting for Dr. Meneely's arrival. Usually at a few minutes after 1:00 P.M., he walked briskly down the center aisle, entered a side door leading to the stage, walked across the stage, and sat in a chair behind the podium for a few moments, saying nothing. After pausing, he rose, cleared his throat, and mounted the podium. He would have done exactly the same thing if the auditorium had been filled.

Meneely stood several feet above floor level. The three of us sat in the chairs on the front row. In order to see Meneely we had to lean back and put our heads on the backs of the folding chairs. This view elongated Meneely into a giant Buddha figure hovering above us. The setup reminded me of Orson Welles at his most extreme weight. Meneely's position directly above us made us slant our bodies into a nearly supine position in our chairs.

Meneely cleared his throat and began. "Welcome to the statistics program for this summer. Those of you among us for the first time will need to know a bit about our course outline." Meneely went on to tell us the lecture schedule and some dates when he would be out of town. He continued, "Aaah, a few housekeeping details before I launch into the agenda for this afternoon's material. I will expect 100 percent attendance at these lectures. You will find the material at times difficult and at times even beyond your grasp. From time to time, I will enter-tain questions, but as a matter of course I ask that the audience hold their questions so that others may follow the flow of my concepts without interruption . . ." He was reading from his notes and did not deviate even one word. This went on three afternoons a week, always immediately following lunch. Staying awake was a constant battle.

There was one memorable day in late June. As usual, Meneely's eyes had become fixed on the ceiling. He was gone—oblivious to anyone's presence. Soon he was lost in statistics, figures, standard deviations of the mean, coefficients of variation, sum of the squares of the differences from the mean . . . and then the sounds began to blur. The sounds came in and out of my mind and resonated with the huge window fans making their futile effort to remove the heat from the unused and un-air-conditioned auditorium. The sounds blended into one sonorous hum and combined with my full stomach to form some unknown sedative compound. A great sense of relaxation and a need for deep sleep overpowered my feeble effort to remain awake. I felt like I had been premedicated for surgery. The muffled sounds, the hum and drone eventually took over, and I slept.

Suddenly a loud bang jerked me to full consciousness. It took a few moments to know what was going on. Hank, long gone into deep sleep, had slipped off the edge of his chair. The folding metal chair had collapsed and fallen backward, making a loud racket. Hank was lying on the floor. He was pitiful. Still barely emerging from coma, he looked like someone who had just had electroshock treatment. He had slobbered down his face, his eyes were bloodshot, his hair all rumpled. He was soaked in sleep sweat. John and I, not in much better shape, pulled the chair back up and then helped Hank get back into a sitting position. All the time, we were looking up at the stage to see if Meneely had noticed. Dr. Meneely paused briefly, looked down at us over the rim of his reading glasses, said nothing, and returned to his lecture and oblivion. He never mentioned the episode to us.

Three days a week, immediately following lunch, we suffered these one-hour lectures. He was obviously using notes from some better-attended class he had taught previously and frequently. Each day we fought the battle to stay awake, and each day one or more of us fell asleep, no matter how hard we tried to stay awake.

As we accumulated more and more data from the experiments, we spent more time in Dr. Meneely's office going over the results. These were the days before computers, so we had to do all our figures by hand or with a mechanically cranked adding machine. It was slow, tedious arithmetic, and Meneely directed us in all the calculations personally. The banter and side remarks and telephone interruptions made the experience delightful. I came to enjoy Meneely's company thoroughly.

George Meneely was a wonderful character. When he was not standing at a podium during the very formal and strange presentations in the theater, he was full of stories. He had traveled extensively, serving on many international research commissions. He seemed to know just about everybody in academic medicine, and would not hesitate to pick up the phone and call them. One time we got into a discussion about Prinzmetal angina—a peculiar set of findings on EKGs associated with anginal chest pain. Meneely's assistant was named Con. He called out, "Con, get Prinzmetal on the phone." In a moment, Meneely was on the phone.

"Myron, George Meneely here. Fine . . . yes . . . no . . . yes . . . no . . . in Chicago. OK." He went on for some time discussing an upcoming meeting.

"Say Myron, when the ST segment is elevated only in the lateral leads with no reciprocal lowering in the limb leads, what do you say to that finding?" He went on into considerably more detail in his questions, losing me in the complexity. Then he hung up. The information was condensed and presented to us, straight from the horse's mouth of Myron Prinzmetal himself. It was as though he had called Pasteur or Lister or even Osler. Here we were in the back end of a rambling VA hospital listening to Meneely talk with the great medical minds of the day. He did that with several other medical luminaries, impressing us with each phone call or side story or tale of some patient he had seen.

Once we were discussing the day's work in his office, and Meneely was playing with a small oddly shaped glass, passing it from one hand to another. I asked him what it was. Without pausing he answered in his most offhand manner, like a stage aside, "Cupping glass. King Farouk's personal physician gave it to me." He continued with what he had been talking about as though this was just a trivial comment. King Farouk had just been deposed as King of Egypt and was a big item in the news.

I could not let it pass and questioned him about the cupping glass.

"Cupping glasses were used by physicians of old. Still use them in Egypt. Ali Hamid Cussef, personal physician to King Farouk, gave me these. Said he often cupped the king with these to reduce fever. Odd ducks, those Egyptian physicians." He described how the hollow cup is first heated and then held tightly on the skin of the patient. The warm air contracts as it cools, sucking skin up into the cup. It was one of many false side tracks that medicine had taken through the centuries. Apparently, it was still a practice in Egypt.

Twice when Hank's car wouldn't run at all, Meneely gave us a ride home. He drove a small foreign car, of all things. I could barely fit into the front seat with him. Hank and John sat in the back. Meneely talked incessantly, one story after another ranging from foreign medical practices, to the social whirl of Nashville, to the eating habits of the natives of Guam, to electrophysiology, and—most often—to his favorite subject, "whole body potassium." Years later he built and operated the first whole body radiation counter. He did some of the first experiments counting the amount of naturally occurring radioactive potassium and calculating the amount of whole body potassium. Meneely would have made a wonderful seventeenth-century scientist. He was fascinated by all aspects of biology and loved inventions. His interests had no bounds, and his laboratory reflected his broad interests.

The life that included the coaches at the Phi Chi house was in sharp contrast to my daytime life at the research lab with Meneely. The coaches had only three interests: sports, beer, and women.

That summer broke all heat records, and for several weeks the temperature had hovered at just over 100 degrees. There was no air conditioning, only rotating fans. Jean and I would hose down the sides of the house each evening, hoping the evaporation might cool down the inside a bit. I could not tell much difference. Each afternoon when I drove up with Hank, the coaches had gathered on the front porch, beers in hand. With the heat so intense, they had stripped off most of their clothes.

Jack, clearly the self-appointed ring leader, was down to jockey shorts, silk socks up to mid-calf, and two-tone brown and white wing-tip shoes. He would stand on the concrete ledge that formed the edge of the front porch, beer in one hand, waving at passing cars on the nearby street. By the time I got to the house in the late afternoon, Jack and the cluster of coaches were drunk. They would be dead drunk by bedtime. Jack, who had a tremendous capacity for booze, would return from dinner, continue drinking, and most nights show up with a different woman. The record player would be blaring one of Johnny Ray's new recordings. It was like living upstairs over a bad nightclub.

Jack waved as I walked up the sidewalk approaching the house. "Hey, Doc, make any discoveries today?" I had made the mistake of telling them about my summer research work. I wished I had never mentioned it. Jack turned to the group who formed his daily audience.

"Doc, here, is doing cancer research. You know, gonna find a cure for it. Putting dogs to sleep. That sorta thing. Tell 'em 'bout your work. Like you told me." It was obvious he was fishing for a straight line and a laugh.

I mumbled something and stood around with the coaches for a while. I never knew what to do. I could feel my face warm up, and I knew it was turning red. Most times I would force a grin and say nothing.

"Hell, I coach ball all year. Teach a little physics and civics back home," Jack said one day. He had a curiously refined manner of holding his little finger delicately off the beer can as he took a swig. He hitched his jockey shorts up a bit, stuck one leg straight out to help with the adjustment, and scratched himself. All of the coaches had fulminant cases of jock itch.

Jack went on. "Another summer and I'm gonna have me a master's degree and eight hundred more a year. This ain't no bad life here, either. Great bunch here," he motioned to the group of coaches. "Away from the old lady all summer. Not bad at all."

Anything was good for a laugh. One of the coaches would whirl around and call out, "whoa," whenever Jack hit a punch line. Another raised his beer can in a toast toward Jack as he laughed.

Jack went on, "Doc, you got it made. Few more years and you got a license to steal." The group laughed again and looked down at the floor. They shook their heads in disbelief. Sometimes Jack was just too much for them.

Being uneasy with this direction of the conversation, I tried to change the subject. "What courses do you take?" I asked.

Jack squatted, did a few deep knee bends, and rotated one leg out to the side to self-adjust his jockey shorts. He looked like a quarterback who couldn't decide whether to pass or run. Any question took a lot of physical preparation and a swig or two of beer. Jack stood up straight, hands on his hips, and faced the street and neighborhood. The group waited patiently. I could imagine Jack in the locker room at half-time. I bet he was hell, especially if his team was down.

"Doc, I'm gonna be straight with you. I take as damn little as I can in school and as much as I can get at night." The group roared approval. As if to settle their laughing, they stood, walked around in little circles, shook their heads, looked back at Jack, laughed again, and finally sat back down on the porch. Jack's really good lines brought on exactly the same ritualized activity from the other coaches. They reminded me of dogs walking around in little circles before lying down.

With the slightest lull in the conversation, I eased off to my room upstairs. It was the same almost every afternoon, except on the weekends, when the coaches drove back to their homes.

There was a wide gulf between the coaches and me. Most of the time they left me uneasy or embarrassed. Yet, in another way, I enjoyed their banter and even envied their free lifestyle. It was certainly in sharp contrast to my life in medical school. There wasn't a phony bone in the group and no pretense of being anything but what they were. However bad or good they were as coaches, it would have been interesting to watch them in a physics or civics class.

The summer with the coaches was my first encounter with feelings of separation. The freshman year in medical school had completely removed all the students from the world around us. The distance we had moved that year was partly responsible for the feelings I had standing around with the coaches. I was physically there, listening, even laughing at their raw humor, but at the same time I was at some distance, detached. The paths we were taking diverged. There is a kind of detachment that is essential for the practice of medicine, and I was experiencing the early phases of that separation. The crucial emotional

detachment of a physician is one reason why it is not wise for physicians to treat close friends or family. I did not realize it at the time, but
I would soon understand that physicians are put in positions apart
from the rest of the world by the people in that other world. It's as if
physicians must somehow be set aside, never fully a part of the world
around them. I experienced those feelings that summer for the first
time with the coaches.

One day at the end of the summer, the coaches loaded their things
into cars and drove off yelling at each other and waving back at Jean
and me. We stood on the porch and waved back to them. Jean said,
"Well at least they paid the rent for the summer, and we made a little
bit for the house on the side."

The summer ended. The faint hint of light brown in the trees,
which had always suggested the upcoming football season, now told
me that the second year of medical school was soon to start. It was a
good feeling, and I was ready.

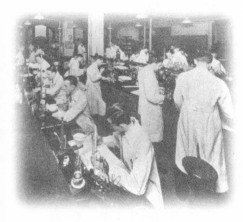

8

A Surgeon in Pathologist's Clothing

21. General and Special Pathology. — Various phases of general and special pathology are presented by lectures, demonstrations, discussions, and laboratory work. Both the gross and the microscopic lesions characteristic of various diseases are studied and correlated. The class attends and may assist with the post mortem examinations performed during the year.

Seventeen hours of lectures and laboratory work a week during the first trimester and fifteen hours of lectures and laboratory work a week during the second trimester of the second year.

Catalogue for 1952–1953
School of Medicine
Vanderbilt University

THE GENTLE COOL WINDS OF EARLY FALL ALTERNATED with the residual hot air of summer. It was a time of transition. We would move from the world of the normal to the world of the abnormal. Pathology was the main course of the second year, and Dr. John Shapiro was its absolute master.

After our summer alone with the coaches, Jean and I were delighted to have the old crew back. Wally, back from his summer on an Indian reservation, was entering his junior year, and he brought with him another year's worth of advice and dire warnings. Oscar had returned from a summer on his farm in Arkansas. Jean had run the children's day camp all summer. Hank, John, and I had finished the drug experiments at the VA, and would have a paper to publish out of that work.

It was the first Friday night dinner of the new semester at the Phi Chi house. All the regulars had gathered, as well as two upcoming freshmen. It was time to summon forth the spirits of those absent.

First came Oscar's mother, reassuringly present after a summer's absence, in fine form in her weekly letter:

Dear Oscar,

I hope you got the cookies I mailed. Tell Wally he can have only two. And tell Jean and Clifton I want them to have some of the cookies, too.

I am glad you have finished all that cutting up bodies. I hope you won't have to do that again. I forgot what you told me you would be studying this year, but maybe it won't be as hard as last year.

Mr. Lewis called from the farm after you left, and said the lame horse is better and that he would antifreeze the toilets before it freezes this fall.

I better close now and go do my grocery shopping. You should get your laundry box soon.

Love,
Mom

Oscar faked reluctance and passed his mother's cookies around, screaming at Wally when he tried to take three.

Then it was time for Wally to do a summoning of his own . . . the "spirit of those to come." Wally began the evocation of Dr. John Shapiro. Shapiro had served as a battalion surgeon in the Italian campaign in World War II and was severely wounded. He nearly died and was left with a protracted infection of the knee joint. The resulting chronic infection left Shapiro with a fused right knee and a low-grade anger at himself and everybody around him. Physically prevented from continuing the rigors of his surgical training, Shapiro had turned

to pathology as an alternative career. The deep forces of psychic fierceness that drive surgeons to do what they do now redirected itself into
an obsession in Shapiro. He would, by God, teach each and every
medical student everything there was to know about human pathology.
It was his divine calling.

Dr. Shapiro had a completely stiff right leg. His knee was frozen
and immobile. When he walked, he had to swing the right leg out in a
wide circle, rise up on the left toes, and then plunk the right foot down
with some force. The sound of his walk struck terror in all sophomore
medical students, like hearing some peg-legged demented sea captain
coming on deck. We could hear him coming long before he appeared.
The wide swing of his right leg made walking along by his right side
impossible; if anyone dared, he would just kick them without missing
a step.

Shapiro was a modern-day Captain Ahab, and his white whale was
any sign of incompetence or shirking in a medical student. He
demanded performance and hard work. He did not tolerate poor
preparation for a lesson. He held nothing back with his tirades and
insults. Lying or trying to fake an answer was unthinkable, and those
few who tried would draw a blistering assault.

Whenever Wally told one of his Shapiro stories, he stood and
walked around the room so he could imitate the limp, which he exaggerated until he got big laughs. Wally should have been on the stage.
That first Friday back at school, Wally chose to tell one of his favorite
Shapiro stories.

One of Wally's classmates was the son of a prominent alumnus of
the medical school. Like many sons of famous fathers, he was directed
by his father's force. The response to this paternal force can take two
directions: It can guide the son in the direction of the father; or, as in
the case of this student, it can drive him in the opposite direction,
perhaps unconsciously provoking the wrath of the father. In either
case, the goal seems to be to get the attention of the father, good or
bad. This student was goofing off, not studying, not answering questions in class, and doing just about everything possible to irritate the

faculty. If it had not been for his father's influence, the student would have been asked to leave in the first year. Shapiro spotted the problem and addressed it directly.

Wally played out the whole scene with his usual exaggerations. Imitating Shapiro, Wally said, "Mr. Smart Ass, please come down in front of the class." Wally walked around in circles, swinging his leg widely and slamming it to the floor. "Mr. Smart Ass, you will leave this class immediately and go home. I am going to give you one day. When you have thought about your life and you have figured out whether you want to be a doctor or not, then you can return to my office and tell me what you have decided. If you decide to study medicine, fine. If you decide to dig ditches, fine. Do you understand me? Are there any questions in that idiotic head of yours?"

The student returned the next day, told Dr. Shapiro that he indeed wanted to study medicine, and began to apply himself. Dr. Shapiro never harassed the student again. In later years the student went on to become a fine surgeon, outdistancing his father's accomplishments.

For all of Shapiro's fierceness, and at times what appeared to be meanness or even cruelty, we all knew he was accurate in what he said. Above all, he was fair and played no favorites. He never said anything he did not mean, and he never withheld his opinions about poor performance. Instilling fear was a part of the man as it was in many of the faculty members of that era. Somehow we knew with certainty that he had our best interests and medicine's best interest deep in his soul. I have never had a professor before or since who commanded that level of respect.

At the heart of everything in pathology was the autopsy—the final arbiter of medicine, the last court of diagnostic appeal, the final answer. Out of the autopsy came the truth of clinical medicine, and Shapiro was the deliverer of those truths. No clinician could hide from its findings, Shapiro made sure of that. The autopsy was also the hub of the course in pathology. Nearly 90 percent of deaths in the hospital came to autopsy, so over the course of a year, we would see the full range of clinical medicine that came to death.

As part of pathology, Shapiro had us take autopsy call, again in groups of four. The residents in pathology did all of the autopsies as soon as possible so that the body could be quickly released to the funeral home. As in physiology lab, each of the four students had an assigned job, which we rotated for each autopsy. One of us did the dissection at the table with the pathology resident. One of us kept notes on the autopsy findings, recording weights of organs, measurements, and descriptions called out by the resident or faculty member. Another student plowed through the clinical chart and abstracted the case into its medical history, physical exam findings, laboratory findings, and the course in the hospital leading up to the point of death. As in physiology, the autopsy team also had scut boys, but there was a big difference between the physiology scut boy and the autopsy scut boy. The autopsy scut boy was the ultimate low man on the totem pole. He had to wash and clean the intestines in a large stainless steel sink, and then clean up the autopsy table when the case was finished. Opening and cleaning the intestines usually took two students.

One night Dr. Shapiro himself showed up to do an autopsy with the resident. He did that often and unexpectedly, just to keep us all on our toes. This happened on one of Wally's autopsies, and it was one of Wally's favorite stories. He told it at least a dozen times.

Wally and a classmate were at the sink in the autopsy room cleaning out the intestines. The sink was filled with the twenty or more feet of intestine. The gut has to be cut with scissors down the entire length and then washed out segment by segment. It is all extremely slippery and therefore nearly impossible to hold, like trying to get a grip on Jell-O. About the time they had finished washing out the length of the gut, a foot or two of the intestine was sucked down the drain.

Wally went into his act, recalling the horror of the night. "I was standing there with my buddy trying to get the intestine back up out of the sink drain. The more we pulled, the more the intestine slipped away down the drain. Hell, it was like trying to hang onto okra or rhubarb. Talk about frantic." Wally was now on his feet. The dining room table was the sink, and his napkin was the tail of the intestines as he feigned pulling at them.

"I was pushing and shoving to get at the intestine. We started to talk in a louder and louder whisper. No matter how hard we tried to grab, the more the gut slipped away. All twenty-one feet. Down the drain. Gone. And with Shapiro right there in the room."

Wally plopped backward into his chair, spent, mouth open in horror. "We began to whisper to each other and huddled over the sink. I could see my whole career following the gut. I had visions of being dismissed on the spot. Talk about spazzed." Wally would imitate the desperation, each time doing it differently depending on the audience.

"My buddy finally whispered to me, 'OK. Who's going to tell the old son of a bitch?' We turned, and there was Shapiro directly behind us, glaring. Somehow the bastard had slipped up on us. Just stood there. We didn't say a word. He didn't say a word. Just shook his head, turned on his good leg, and clomped back to the autopsy table. Then he stopped and wheeled around and said, 'Oh, by the way, tell your friend I'm not old.' He never said another word about the missing intestines."

In addition to our other lectures, Shapiro scheduled three special sessions a week with Dr. Ernest Goodpasture. Dr. Goodpasture was and still is one of the deities of Vanderbilt School of Medicine. He uncovered the first method to culture viruses by planting them on chick embryos and then sealing the egg. He wrote the first book on a systematic pathological study of a variety of viruses. Prior to Goodpasture's work, viruses were considered to be a mysterious element that could pass through ordinary filter paper. In fact they were called "filterable infectious agents" before they were called viruses. All that we know about viruses stems from work that followed Goodpasture's monumental original work. Many scientists believed that Goodpasture should have received the Nobel Prize for his research. Shapiro believed that and more. In Shapiro's mind, Goodpasture was God's directly appointed Saint of Pathology. Shapiro adored and worshipped him. He expected and demanded that we follow suit, and he had a method to ensure that we did.

Dr. Goodpasture was Shapiro's opposite in nearly all aspects. He spoke in a very soft voice and looked like Clarence the angel in the perennial Christmas movie "It's a Wonderful Life." He was kind, gentle, and extremely polite.

Dr. Goodpasture had a routine and a system to his lectures. He lectured a bit, and then he had students stand and answer his questions about the day's topic. The subjects were posted well ahead of time—Dr. Shapiro made sure of that. We were expected to read the material before we attended Goodpasture's lectures, and there had just better not be a question we could not answer. Dr. Goodpasture had a roll-call book of our class, and he went strictly down the alphabet. He usually quizzed two or three students per session. We had committed the alphabetical listing of our class to memory, so we could predict within one or two lectures when we would be called on, so we could cram for the session.

As if the rigor of facing Dr. Goodpasture, the world's greatest living pathologist, were not enough, there was Shapiro's close scrutiny, which brought fear and terror into the process. Like guards in a maximum security prison, Shapiro, the junior faculty, and the pathology residents sat on the back row of the lecture room with the entire class in front of them. Shapiro carefully monitored in detail our responses to Goodpasture's quizzing. Any wrong answer brought an audible outburst from Shapiro. Hank devised the Shapiro Scale of Loathing and Disgust for Bad Student Answers.

The first level of disapproval on Hank's Shapiro Scale, usually in response to a minor incomplete answer, was a quiet, "Good God A'mighty!" His second level of disapproval, to a more serious omission of knowledge, was, "Oh, Hell. Damn. A fool would know that." The third level, usually when a major part of the correct answer was missing, was a fairly loud, "Damn. Hell fire. You are a stupid idiot." The highest level of damnation, reserved for overtly incorrect answers, was a shuffling of his bad leg, stamping of his good foot, and all sorts of combinations of "Damn," "Hell," and even "Shit." The "F" word was just not permissible in 1952, or Shapiro would probably have thrown in a few of those to boot.

During one of my times to stand and be quizzed by Dr. Goodpasture, I stumbled on some detail about cartilage formation. I vividly recall the blood rushing to my head as I heard sounds from the back of the room. After the session, I asked Hank what score I made on his Shapiro Scale. Hank said it was not repeatable in polite company.

Although death occurs at any time, it seemed that nearly every autopsy call came at night. No matter where we were or what we were doing, we had to go to the hospital if our four-man team was up for call. I did not realize it then, but this was our introduction to learning that medicine and its demands came first, no matter what. Taking autopsy call was the first part of a slow progression into the demands of medicine. It was also one more step away from the world outside of medicine. As I now look back on the experiences, the study of medicine moved us year by year into a very isolated world, removed from nearly all social contact outside of our little circle of classmates and our patients.

In addition to lectures and our afternoon microscope laboratory sessions, we met each week for a whole morning to review the previous week's autopsy findings. Shapiro was in command, and we were his crew. Our entire class filed into the autopsy room and mounted three unusual metal racks. They looked like distorted jungle gyms or climbing equipment from playgrounds. Each row on the rack had three metal bars: one bar to sit on, one bar as a hand rail in front, and a third rail below for foot support. They were uncomfortable beyond description, especially after a couple of hours. About six students could sit on each row, eighteen to the rack. One rack of students was placed in front of the autopsy table, with one rack on each end of table. Shapiro and the residents, all in white gowns and gloves, stood in a row behind the metal autopsy table, surrounded by the rising ranks of fifty-two medical students, when a class was full. In our white coats we were sailors hanging on yardarms, looking down at officers on the deck of some very strange sailing vessel. The scene was as old as medical science, and reminded me of paintings of early surgeons in amphitheaters demonstrating dissections to huddled medical students. This added a mystique that we were always seeking.

Some long-forgotten student had aptly dubbed the weekly sessions "organ recitals." Several large ceramic pots filled with organs sat on the metal autopsy table. Each pot contained the organs from an autopsy. Dr. Shapiro would then read the number of the autopsy, never the patient's name. With that clue, the four students who had participated in the autopsy filed down to one end of the table and stood at full attention facing Shapiro. One student read the clinical summary, first giving the patient's history, the findings, the course in the hospital, and the terminal clinical events. Then Dr. Shapiro would pull one organ after another out of the ceramic pot. In a few moments all the organs were displayed on the table, oriented from head to toes, forming a peculiar homunculus . . . lungs, heart, liver, intestines, kidneys, and internal genitalia. Laid out that way, we got a quick look at all the vital organs. It struck me how small the internal vital machinery really is, at least compared to the bulk of a human body.

Shapiro called on each of the four students who had done the autopsy. He questioned them about the findings of the autopsy until the details were clearly laid out in a logical and understandable fashion. We would then hear and see how the findings at autopsy correlated with the clinical findings before death. We could look at the diseased heart valves and see the defect that generated the murmur recorded in the medical record. We could see the metastases of the cancer now replacing the normal liver tissue. We would see the obstructed ureters dilated to near garden-hose size, causing hugely bloated and failed kidneys.

These were magical times for me. Shapiro made the study of disease come alive. If there was a clinical finding, there was a pathological explanation. There was never a day for me without sheer fascination and wonder. We learned that a careful history and physical exam combined with a careful choice of lab tests could, in most cases, lead to very accurate diagnoses. We learned that in the face of a quick death or an absent history, there would be little correlation between the clinical course and the findings at autopsy. The history and story of the patient were as vital then as they always will be.

Of all my professors, Shapiro remains most vivid in my mind. There was one trait that did not come out during his course, and that was a visible measure of his heart. As soon as the course in pathology was completed, that very day, Shapiro called me "Clifton" as I passed him in the hall. I was no longer "Mister Meador." I felt a deep glow of acceptance and achievement. I knew immediately I had passed his course. It was Shapiro's way of telling us. He had accepted me into his ranks, as he did for all but one of our class.

We progressed into the next phase of studying medicine.

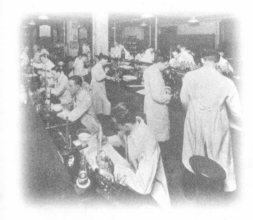

9

HARPER'S BIZARRE

Students who have had no reported failures may be required to withdraw from the school if their work has been of a generally unsatisfactory quality.

Catalogue for 1952–1953
School of Medicine
Vanderbilt University

MADISON HARPER APPEARED IN THE AFTERNOON pathology lab one day, several weeks after the beginning of our sophomore year. For several days we thought he was a new member of the pathology faculty, or maybe a visiting professor. His much older age and unusual accent threw us off. He sounded like an old, hesitant Englishman who'd had too much to drink. Harper often walked up and down the long lab tables where we were studying our microscope slides. Occasionally he would say something like, "Aah, good job there, old chap." "Old chap" was his standard greeting.

After about a week we figured out that Harper was not faculty, but a thirty-eight-year-old transfer student coming into our class. Soon after that we figured out why his accent sounded so strange. It was a complete affectation. Harper had grown up in Chicago.

Hank discovered that Harper had transferred from some school in Vienna. Harper called himself "Maddie," short for Madison, but we soon dubbed him "Harpo" after one of the Marx brothers.

In our lectures, when he chose to show up, he sat next to Walter. Walter had moved into the Phi Chi house and had become a regular member of our group. Walter soon became the unofficial biographer of Harper. His interest stemmed not from like or dislike of Harper; rather, Walter saw his subject as a fascinating enigma worthy of close observation and frequent reports at supper. Walter got a lot of mileage out of the stories, and soon stories of Harper began to take a place beside Oscar's mother's letters from home and Wally's forbidding descriptions of faculty yet-to-come. Each Friday night the documented Harpo observations were reported, with additional data from others submitted.

Walter quickly realized that the more he studied Harper, the more he was rewarded with distinguishing features. Besides the fake accent, there was the harsh tweed jacket and nearly matching trousers. Even more notable, Walter noticed pajama sleeves sticking out of the coat and pajama bottoms sticking out of Harper's trouser legs. We were skeptical on the first report, but sure enough, there they were. When Walter asked him why he wore the pajamas all the time, Harper answered, "You see old chap, my woolens are from the Outer Hebrides. They itch terribly. Hence my need for the pajamas as undergarments."

Harper was as distinguishable by what he carried as what he wore. He always carried a large stack of dog-eared papers under one arm and several books under the other. He somehow dangled his wooden microscope case on two fingers beneath the reams of paper. The rest of us kept our microscopes in lockers in the pathology lab. Harper, for reasons unknown, chose to carry his from class to class.

In the midst of his bundle of papers was a number of photographs of Harper's new bride. Apparently, Harper had married just before returning to the states, leaving his new bride in Vienna. The photos showed his bride in all states of dress and undress. Her pose in most of the pictures was highly suggestive. In some she was downright porno-graphic. Harper delighted in passing the photos around for all of us to see. In many lectures, you could see one photograph after another being passed row to row throughout the lecture. Harper would stand at the end of the lecture and ask for everyone to turn in the photographs. He seemed quite proud of the pictures and, without any hesitation, pulled them out if requested.

Harper seemed unaware or unconcerned with most any rule of polite or expected behavior, whether it be in his relations with other students or with the school.

Walter had noticed that Harper constantly looked at Walter's notes during lectures, obviously copying them. Harper's own notes showed a strange pattern. There was writing on the left side of the page, then a large blank space, and then writing on the right side of the page. Walter sat on Harper's right and kept his left arm across his notes as a matter of habit. Walter's arm obscured the notes down the middle of the left page. No problem. Harper just copied what he could see and left blank what he could not see. After class he would ask Walter for the notes so he could fill in the blank spaces. Walter sneaked some of Harper's notes and passed them along with the photos so we could all see the bizarre pattern.

Although he was a sophomore, Harper did not restrict himself to second-year classes or labs. One day he would be on rounds with the junior students in medicine. The next day he would join a group of seniors in the pediatrics clinic. He even spent time with the freshmen in the cadaver lab. Within a few weeks, everyone in medical school knew him and had a story to tell. He had showed up in nearly every class or clinic or ward rounds from the freshman through the senior classes. He had free rein of the entire medical school. We were amazed that the faculty had not addressed his chaotic behavior.

Their lack of action certainly did not derive from lack of notice. Harper's behavior was conspicuous on all fronts and to all viewers, to teachers as well as classmates.

One day in class a professor had presented a case of chronic, protracted fever or what is called FUO, for "fever of unknown origin." The professor was calling on students by name from his roll book.

"Mister Harper, what do you say?" the professor asked.

"Poor chap, died of a ruptured aortic aneurysm," Harper answered without even looking up from the book he was reading.

It was as far off and far out as an answer can get. The differential diagnosis for an FUO includes all kinds of obscure infections, with tuberculosis high on the list. Then there are long lists of rare diseases also associated with protracted fever. Vascular accidents are not on the list by any stretch of the imagination. The professor paused, looked perplexed, even quizzical like he had misunderstood the answer. There were scattered giggles from the class.

"Pardon, I'm not sure I heard you," prompted the professor. He was one of the physicians in town who volunteered his time, so he did not know one of us from the other. He had no way of knowing of Harper's growing reputation for inappropriate answers and behavior.

"No bother, really, old chap," Harper responded with some anima-tion. "You see, the poor chap died of a ruptured aortic aneurysm." Harper was quite certain by his tone of voice. He often gave answers that did not resemble the question asked, and he always did it in a loud, assertive voice.

The professor, whom we had only seen once before, was obviously puzzled. He did not, however, want to jump too quickly to the obvious conclusion that Harper was out of his mind. "Anyone else think this man has a ruptured aneurysm?"

The giggles spread across the classroom. No one raised a hand. The professor went on to the next name on the list, ignoring Harper for the rest of the session.

Even when he vanished altogether, Harper still managed to do so in a manner that confused and bewildered.

One of his conspicuous absences occurred soon after Dean Youmans decided to add field trips during the second year. The idea was that we should move out from the fixed curriculum and get a broader view of our roles as physicians and medical leaders. In the 1950s, many county boards of health were identical with the county medical societies, so it fell to physicians across much of the country to administer and monitor all public health programs. We were to make day-long field trips to a sewage disposal plant, a meat packing plant, a county health department, and a water treatment facility. Since only a few students had cars, we had to rely on the town students to borrow family cars and drive us to the locations. Harper loved the field trips and was usually in the center of the group surrounding our guides, who were workers from the various locations. At the sewage disposal plant, we followed the flow of sewage from its raw stages to its ultimate purification and removal. As the plant operator said, "At that stage, the bacterial count is no higher than in peanut butter." That put the quietus on peanut butter for a while for me.

At the end of the visit to the sewage plant, we loaded back into our ride groups and headed back to the medical school. Harper had switched riding groups, but no one else knew it. He was inadvertently left at the sewage disposal plant, about twenty miles out in the most rural part of the county. The class discovered the next day what had happened. We waited one day, then another, and then a third. On the fourth day, Harper showed up in class. Even Walter could not find out what had happened to him. Harper never commented on his disappearance, nor did he seem in the least upset by being left in the country with no ride.

Anticipation quickly built over the first direct encounter between Harper and Shapiro. Harper, being in the H's, had not yet been called on by Goodpasture. His four-man autopsy team had not yet done an autopsy. We had overheard the residents talking about Shapiro's opinion of Harper. All they said was that Shapiro had figured that Harper was not your usual medical student. The first live encounter finally came at an organ recital session in the autopsy room. Dr. Shapiro pulled an entire colon out onto the dissecting table. He slid it around until he had exposed the entire lining of the colon. The mucosa was black, like it had been coated with soot.

He wheeled on his good leg toward Harper. Harper was sitting on the third metal row, huddled with all of his papers, books, and his microscope case.

"Mr. Harper, tell the class what you think about this colon." Shapiro held the colon up for all to see the black lining.

Harper didn't hesitate. "Obvious case of suicide. Poor chap did himself in." Harper answered in his usual self-assured tone.

The class roared with laughter. We knew about *melanosis coli*, a condition caused by chronic laxative abuse, where somehow the mucosa of the colon becomes darkly pigmented. It was thought then to be a benign condition only discoverable at autopsy or sometimes by proctoscopy. We had been waiting to see an example ever since we had been told about it in lectures.

Dr. Shapiro could barely contain himself. He seldom smiled—in fact, *never* would be closer to the truth. This time, though, he could not hide his grin. "SUICIDE," he yelled. "Mr. Harper, how in God's name can you come up with suicide?"

"Quite obviously suicide. Poor chap gave himself a sodium hydroxide enema." Harper answered in a tone suggesting impatience.

With that, the class laughed even louder, but there was an undercurrent of anticipation. How would Shapiro, the fierce destroyer of the inept and dismantler of the foolish, handle Madison Harper? Shapiro wheeled on his good leg, swung his stiff leg out widely, and then quickly bumped out of the room, calling back over his shoulder in a barely muffled laugh to the chief resident, "Dismiss the class, that's enough for one day." It was an even stranger response in some ways than Harper's answer.

Shapiro's decision to leave the field rather than dress Harper down struck us as a postponement rather than a result, so we could hardly wait for Harper's autopsy group to report at organ recital. The day finally came, and we figured it would be a delayed reckoning. There were three autopsies to be reported that day. Harper's group was the last of the three. Shapiro had used up all but twenty minutes with the first two cases. Shapiro called out the autopsy number of Harper's case. Three of the team filed down from the metal racks and stood by the table. Shapiro paced up and down behind the table.

Shapiro called out, "Mister Harper, would you give us the pleasure of your company? We are short on time."

Behind me and to my right I saw a white form stand up on the handrail metal bar. Harper looked like a great bird ready to take flight. He leapt—papers, flowing white coat and all—over the row of students in front of him. When he landed on the wet floor, his feet went out, and he slid under the end of the autopsy table. His papers scattered all over the place. The class erupted. The residents turned their backs to hide their laughter. Shapiro just stood there shaking his head. "Mister Harper, please get up off the floor."

Harper stood, drenched from the run-off water from the autopsy table. "Mister Harper," Shapiro finally said after the laughing subsided, "we have only a few minutes left. Please shorten your clinical summary so we can get to the findings of the autopsy."

Harper had been assigned the job of abstracting the clinical summary. He had two choices. He could condense the clinical story, or he could read it as fast as he could. He chose the latter approach. He launched into something that sounded like an auctioneer in a strange accent, reading the clinical summary as fast as his mouth and tongue could move.

Shapiro stood in obvious disbelief, shaking his head slowly. "Mister Harper, stop. Stop now." Harper kept reading. "STOP," Shapiro yelled. Harper stopped.

Shapiro said, "We are out of time. Mister Harper, see me in my office immediately." Once again, the anticipated explosion did not occur. Perhaps Shapiro was just taken off balance; with each encounter, Harper somehow managed to up the absurdity.

Finally, Harpo managed a scene worthy of his Marx brothers–inspired nickname. As the course progressed, Harper's loads of papers, books, and other paraphernalia had increased. It was the day of the final microscopic practical examination in pathology. The long black benches in the student lab were covered by our microscopes, one at each lab site. Under each scope was a slide representing some lesion of an unknown tissue. We were to look at the slide, write down what tissue it was, and what disease process we saw. For example, we might say "adenocarcinoma of the pancreas" or "myocardial infarction" or "glomerulonephritis," or whatever microscopic lesion we saw. When time was called, we would move to the next microscope.

We always waited in the hallway until all of the students were present, then Dr. Shapiro would lead us into the lab and direct us to our designated first station. This day, we waited and we waited. No Harper. Shapiro was pacing back and forth, mumbling to himself. "Has anyone seen Mr. Harper?" he asked in a loud voice.

We waited another minute or two. Suddenly, the double swinging doors at the far end of the long corridor burst open. Here came Harper, at full speed. His right arm was filled with his papers, dog-eared and hanging off at the edges. In his left arm were several books. Attached to his right index finger, barely being grasped, was his wooden microscope case. He looked like some weird and comical cowboy crashing through the saloon doors, looking for a fight. He came forward toward the assembled group, walking as fast as he could.

The student lab was being remodeled, and along the walls of the corridors were several of the old lab benches. There were four legs in the center of each bench, with long unsupported extensions out to each side. Thus, each bench formed a potential see-saw. Were any weight put on one end of the long bench, the other end would shoot up in the air. Harper apparently did not know that.

As he came almost running down the hall, he headed for one of the benches so he could put down some of the extra weight of his accumulated stuff. Someone yelled, "Watch out! Don't do that." It was too late.

Down went his microscope, books, and stacks of papers. Time slowed as we all watched the inevitable—so unpredictable only a moment earlier—occur. Up shot the other end of the long bench, hitting the fire extinguisher lightly attached to the wall above. Down came the newly unmoored fire extinguisher. Out in all directions sprayed the foam from its nozzle after it hit the floor. The class scattered. Shapiro yelled at Harper. Harper dove for the whipping end of the nozzle, and finally bent the hose and stopped the spray. He was drenched in foam. It would be difficult to choreograph a scene of slapstick as effectively as Harper's one-man improv. Again, Shapiro was stymied. He threw up his hands, lacking any comeback. "Let's take an examination," was all he said as he swung open the doors to let us into the lab. As we entered, he just shook his head from side to side, saying nothing.

Somehow Harper survived this fiasco and all his other miscues and oversteps that trimester. He remained in the class until the end of the first term before being dismissed by Dean Youmans. He did not come back. We never knew what happened to him. Someone thought he saw a name like his in a list of people from Minnesota. Someone heard that he had gone to dental school in Oregon. Another thought he had become a pharmacist. But no one knew for sure, and we never heard from Madison Harper again. He was always a mystery. He must have been able to perform at some high level to finish undergraduate school, get admitted to medical school, and then be accepted for transfer. Maybe he could take tests and repeat material in written form. Who knows how he got to where he was. Despite the fact that every student in every class knew of Harper, none of us really knew him in the slightest, not even his biographer, Walter.

There is one observation worth noting about the Harpers of this world. Wherever I have been, no matter how competitive or rarefied the atmosphere, there has always been a Harper, someone who defies all description, is oblivious to his surroundings, makes stupid mistakes, and appears to lack even the most basic components of common sense. They can even be found in some fairly high positions, completely unsuited for what they are doing, out of their league and, as Harper was, nearly oblivious to those around them. Yet, somehow, there they are. I saw Harpers in my residency in New York. I saw them on visits to the National Institute of Health. I have met Harpers as faculty members at several universities where I have made site visits. I saw them in the Army medical corps, once as the commanding officer of a hospital. Although Harper is an extreme case, characters similar to him show up in nearly every medical school every few years.

Somehow, no matter how careful or selective the procedures, there will always be someone who slips through the process. It still surprises me when I encounter one. I always think back to Harper. He will always be my benchmark for someone rising to a level far beyond his competence.

After I finished medical school, I came to know Dr. Shapiro as a colleague, a close friend, and as one of my patients. One day, many years later, he suddenly asked me if I ever understood Madison Harper. I said I did not. He smiled and shook his head in disbelief, still stymied after all those years.

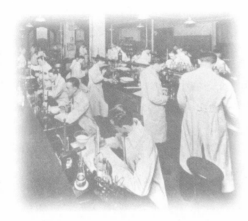

10

SHOES,
WINDOW
SCREENS,
AND MEAT

522. Parasitic Diseases — Diagnostic Laboratory Methods, Clinical Aspects and Control Measures. A course of lectures, demonstrations and laboratory exercises in which the animal parasites of man, their vectors and the diseases which they produce are studied. The biological activities of parasites are emphasized. Patients and case histories are used wherever possible; methods of treatment may be discussed, and prevention and control are stressed. Five hours a week during the second trimester of the second year.

Joint clinics may be held in conjunction with the Department of Medicine for the purpose of integrating the teaching of preventive and clinical medicine. These clinics have not been provided in formal schedule but may be held when patients are admitted to the Hospital suffering from such conditions as typhoid fever, malaria, undulant fever, endemic typhus fever, tularemia, and lead poisoning.

Catalogue for 1952–1953
School of Medicine
Vanderbilt University

PARASITOLOGY DISAPPEARED FROM THE VANDERBILT catalogue course listings the year following the entry above. Our class took the next to last course in parasitology offered at the school. In a few years parasitology would cease to be a course in most medical schools in the United States. It would no longer be necessary. Parasitic diseases—now very rare in the United States—were still present, though in diminishing numbers, in the 1950s, especially in the rural South. The disappearance of parasitic diseases is a story of the extraordinary power of the scientific method in action, coupled with the extreme power of public education. Above all, it is a story of prevention over cure.

The dramatic reduction in the prevalence of parasitic diseases is paralleled by the differences in the amount of written material in the text books then and now. In the 1950 first edition of Harrison's *Principles of Internal Medicine*, there are more than sixty pages devoted to parasitic diseases, making up nearly 4 percent of the whole book. Four entire sections of the book were devoted to the four classes of parasites infesting man. There was a section for protozoans (malaria being one), a section on nematodes (round worms), a section on flukes, and a section on cestodes (tapeworms).

In contrast, the 2002 Fifth Edition of Cecil's *Essentials of Medicine* contains a mere four pages under the title "Infectious Diseases of Travelers; Protozoal and Helminthic Infections." The parasitic diseases are lumped with other diseases that are now limited to third-world and underdeveloped countries. The South of my youth in the 1930s *was* a third-world, underdeveloped country, still suffering the human ravages, destruction, and remnant diseases of the Civil War and the years of federal occupation that followed.

Dr. Alvin Keller, our professor of parasitology, had served as a public health officer in the South in the 1920s and '30s. He had seen the human misery and devastation produced by parasitic diseases and malnutrition. The principle parasitic diseases affecting so much of the rural South were hookworm, round worms, and malaria. There was another pandemic disease of nutritional origin— pellagra. All of these were completely eradicated by the early 1960s. Dr. Keller made the story of the elimination of these diseases vivid and fascinating.

Most parasites are carried in human feces and must be identified in stool specimens. Malaria, an exception, is carried in the blood. It would be our job as clinical clerks in the third year to be able to find and identify all of the North American parasites in the feces of our patients. Stool lab made up half the parasitology course.

Human parasites are highly variable organisms, and they are very different from bacteria. In the first place, parasites are animals; in contrast to bacteria, most of which can be classified as plants. Parasites range from unicellular protozoans, like the malaria parasite, to highly developed worms that can grow to nearly twenty feet long, like the tapeworm. There is something nauseous, bordering on horror, about a worm taking up residence inside the human body. Somehow, that life form is getting too evolved, too close to a higher form of life for comfort. Bacteria are passively swept into our bodies in air or food or water. Parasites, however, especially worms, often have to find us, crawl through our skin, and then burrow inside us. There is a low-grade dread that they are actually stalking us or, worse, that they have some conscious intent to get us. Finally, there is something really unsettling and alien about an infection inside you that can still crawl around. At least bacteria and viruses tend to stay put, once they settle down.

These unsettling thoughts were vividly brought out when I saw pictures of a round worm crawling out of the nose of a little girl, already bloated from combined hookworm, chronic malaria, and malnutrition. Her mother, in her thirties, stood by her side. She was haggard and looked to be in her sixties. Both were barefooted. Walker Evans and James Agee captured similar images of the rural South in their poetic prose and photographic classic, "Let Us Now Praise Famous Men." Nearly a fourth of rural Southerners, black and white alike, had the vicious and lethal combination of all three diseases: hookworm, chronic malaria, and malnutrition.

Evans and Agee were taking their pictures and writing about people who lived in the same section of south Alabama where I grew up. They could just as well have been in my grammar school. I recall coming home one day in the third grade in 1939. I asked my mother why the children who came into town from the country were so pale and yellow, but those of us from town were pink. She thought a minute, with a very sad look on her face. She told me they were poor and did not have food or shoes or clothing like us. She did not know of the pandemic of hookworm or malaria or pellagra, and the resulting anemia that underlay their pallor.

It was only when I learned of the high prevalence of these diseases across the South that I understood what had afflicted so many of my classmates. Dr. Keller made the epidemiological figures vivid when he told stories of families and patients he had treated earlier in his career.

In addition to my epidemiological interest in the diseases, the lives of the parasites themselves fascinated me. Nothing in science fiction can outdo the life cycle of any parasite. Over and over, I was amazed at the complexity of their circuitous lives. I was even more in awe of the many scientists who unraveled these almost unbelievable transformations in life forms. Take, for example, the life of the hookworm, *Ancylostoma duodenale* in the old world and *Necatur americanus* in the new world. These worms, almost a half inch long, are carried in the human intestinal tract, where the worm hooks its mouth parts onto the lining of the intestine and begins to suck blood. Periodically, the worm releases its hold and moves progressively down the intestines. Each adult worm drinks about 0.5 ml of blood a day, or a teaspoon in about ten days. The "disease" produced is an iron deficiency anemia from the blood loss. In children, the anemia is often coupled with malnutrition, and those who survived to puberty often showed delayed physical, mental, and sexual development. In the early 1930s, 36 percent of Southerners, black and white, had hookworm infestations.

The life cycle of the hookworm reads like something from an alien world. The adult female hookworm, after copulation (if you can imagine that!) and fertilization, lays about ten thousand eggs per day. The eggs are discharged, unhatched, with the feces. If the ground conditions are moist, the eggs hatch into larvae after a few days, and in a few more days they are infectious. They lay in wait for any bare feet, burrow into the skin, and then make their way into the blood stream. There is sometimes intense itching of the feet, called "ground itch," in the affected areas. The larvae then find their way to the lungs, where they burrow into the small air sacs. Then they migrate up the trachea into the pharynx and are swallowed. During this phase, the patient may develop a cough. Finally, in three to four weeks, the larvae mature in the intestines, attach, begin to suck blood, and lay eggs. The creepy and bizarre life cycle starts all over.

In addition to hookworm infestation, nearly a third of the inhabitants of the rural South had chronic malaria from living in houses with no window screens. Malaria, a word meaning "bad air," is carried by a mosquito. It produces recurrent chills and fever and great chronic debility. My mother had suffered with chronic malaria for many years of her life, and was partially blind from too much quinine in her youth.

As if malaria and hookworm were not enough, add to those the scourge of malnutrition, specifically in the form of pellagra. About 25 percent of the Southern population had pellagra, a disease caused by lack of tryptophan, an essential amino acid, in the diet. The diet of Southern tenant farmers then consisted almost entirely of corn bread and hog fat belly, neither of which had any significant amount of tryptophan. A deficiency of tryptophan produces pellagra, which is manifested by severe chronic diarrhea and a vicious skin eruption on the exposed body parts. The final phase of pellagra is mental deterioration, dementia, and death.

By the mid-1930s, not only was the source of hookworm known, but equally important, scientists had unraveled the causes and prevention of pellagra and malaria. Through the efforts of the Rockefeller Foundation and the public health departments of the states, a massive education campaign was set into motion. The final result of that campaign was to render the South free of all three of its ravaging diseases: malaria, by controlling mosquito reproduction and screening doors and windows; pellagra, by teaching the need for meat in the diet and by vitamin supplementation; and hookworm, by the wearing of shoes. I don't know of a more dramatic and successful story of the use of science and education to eliminate disease on such a wide scale. The modernization of the South could not have been considered until those three diseases were controlled.

In addition to learning the life cycles and epidemiology of the parasites, we learned to identify the parasites under the microscope. The stool lab sessions in parasitology stood in stark contrast to the fascinating lectures of Dr. Keller. Every Tuesday afternoon, immediately after lunch, we gathered along the long black benches of the student lab. We were to learn to recognize all of the parasites that infested humans, at least those found in feces.

As junior and senior clinical clerks, we would be responsible for examining all stools on every patient we saw. The purpose of the afternoon lab was to teach us how to do that. We would be required to look for and identify all ova and parasites, called "stool for O and P" on the intern's yellow student order sheet. In addition we would test each stool for occult blood. Stool lab, as we called it, became—above all else—a test of our willpower over more visceral reactions.

Some poor soul, somewhere deep in the basement of the medical school, kept each parasite sustained in vats of human feces. Each Tuesday, these large ceramic vats were wheeled into the lab on a large pushcart. One vat was marked "hookworms," another "ascaris" (round worms), another "tenia solium" (human tapeworm), and still another "giardia" ("when available" was taped underneath).

By two o'clock, the odor of the lab (stench is more accurate) was overpowering. It took all the stamina and determination I could muster to stay at my desk looking down into the drop of black fluid spread out on the slide. This put the fecal specimen only a few inches from my nostrils. It was like sticking my head into a cesspool or septic tank. Survive the stool lab, and you could handle nearly any kind of filth and remain functional. The faculty told us over and over that nothing human is repugnant. The stool lab in parasitology was the acid test for that statement.

Gagging was contagious. When a single gag happened, it swept throughout the lab, going out of control within seconds. One gag and then two gags and then three gags, then a whole bench gagging. By that time, one or more students ran to the hallway for some relief and fresh air. No one actually vomited, but some came very close to it. The gagging brought hysterical laughter from the remaining classmates, and then the cycle would repeat itself. Gradually, over the course of several weeks, the gagging ceased as we became more and more immune to the foul smells or wretched appearances of the worms. In addition to learning to deal with an unpleasant task, stool lab gave me great respect for what the preceding scientists had endured in their search for truth about parasites.

Both Dr. Kampmeier, who would teach us physical diagnosis, and Dr. Keller impressed over and over that no disease had ever been eliminated by any treatment. Diseases cannot be eliminated by treatment. The reason is obvious. Until the reservoir of a disease is contained, removed, or barred from human contact, the disease will persist. Treatment is always an action downstream from the cause. Treatment is always an after-the-fact reaction.

I cannot think of a better example of the power of the scientific method, of prevention, and of public education than the story of the unraveling and elimination of parasitic diseases and pellagra from the rural South. No treatment was involved. All it took was wearing shoes, installing window screens, and eating lean meat.

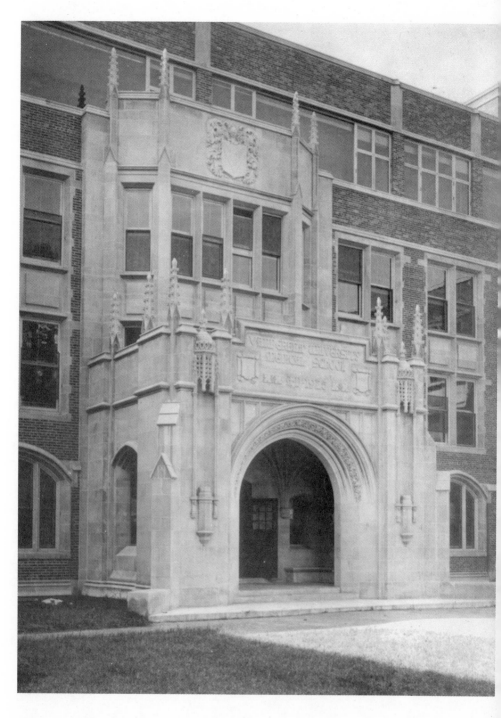

Entrance to Vanderbilt School of Medicine, 1951.

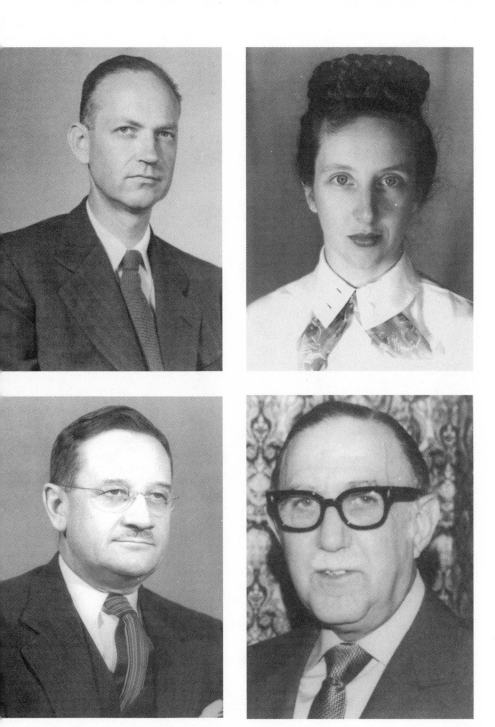

Top left: Dr. James "Jungle Jim" Ward, professor of anatomy. ***Top right:*** Dr. Mildred Stahlman, *professor of pediatrics.* ***Bottom left:*** Dr. Rudolph Kampmeier, professor of medicine. ***Bottom right:*** Dr. Alvin Keller, professor of preventive medicine.

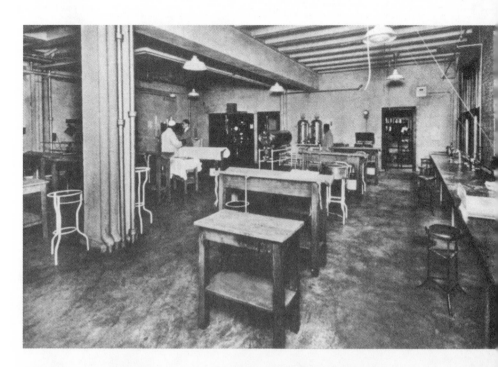

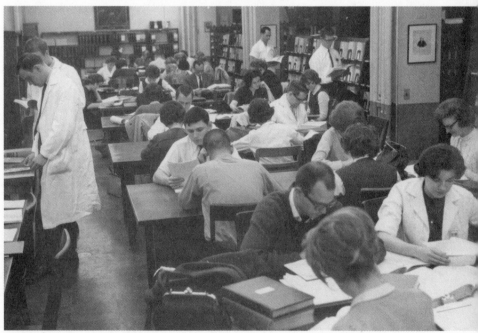

Top: Experimental surgery laboratory. Bottom: Medical and nursing students in the library.

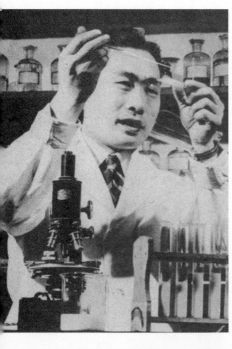
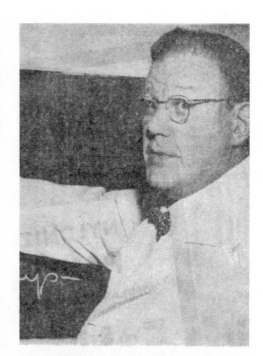
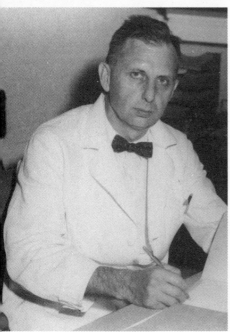
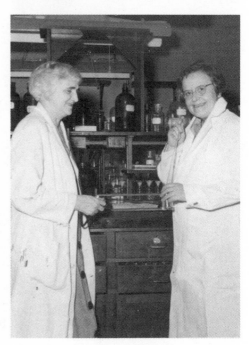

*Top left: Dr. Ray Meng, physiology. **Top right:** Dr. George Meneely, Veterans Administration research laboratory. **Bottom left:** Dr. John Shapiro, professor of pathology. **Bottom right:** Helen Frank (left) and Dr. Ann Minot, clinical chemistry laboratory.*

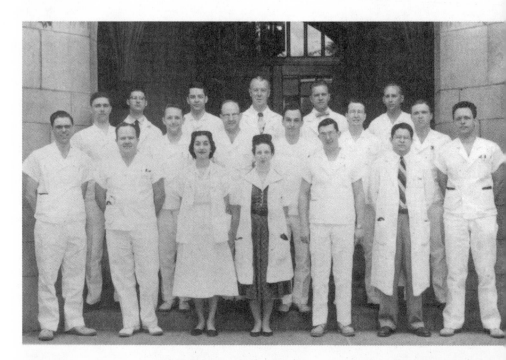

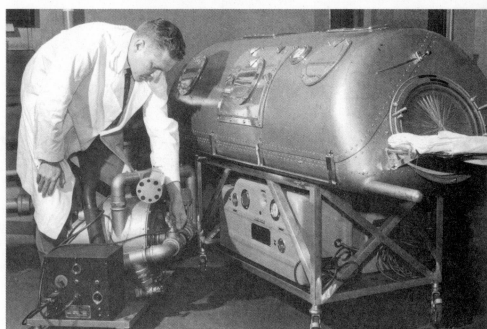

Top: *Department of Pediatrics, five chairmen: Riley (second from right, row 1); Stempfel (third from right, row 1); Merrill (far right, row 2); Denny (far left, back row); and Christie (center, back row).* **Bottom:** *Dr. Randolph Batson and iron lung.*

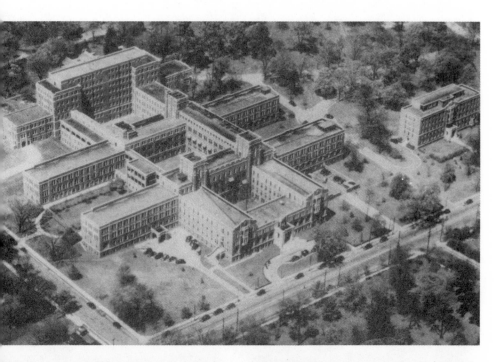

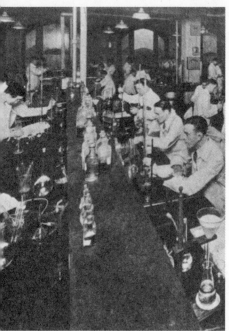
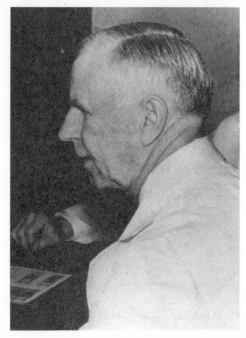

Top: Vanderbilt School of Medicine, hospital, and clinics complex, circa 1940s (left). School of Nursing building (far right). ***Bottom left:*** Freshman biochemistry laboratory. ***Bottom right:*** Dr. Ernest Goodpasture.

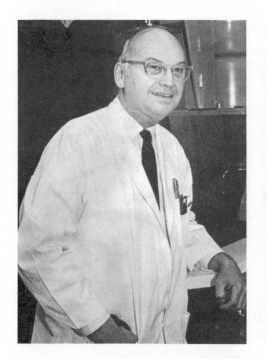
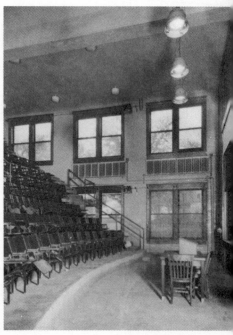
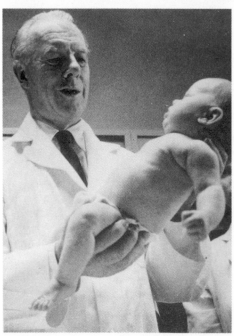
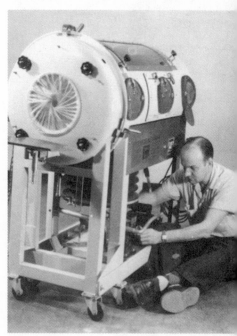

Top left: *Dr. Elliott Newman, professor of medicine and director of the Clinical Research Center.*
Top right: *Old amphitheater.* **Bottom left:** *Dr. Amos Christie, chairman of pediatrics, and baby.*
Bottom right: *Iron lung and technologist.*

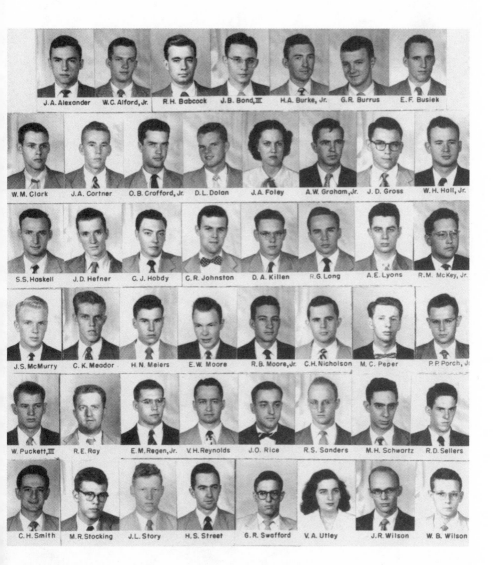

J.A. Alexander W.C. Alford, Jr. R.H. Babcock J.B. Bond, III H.A. Burke, Jr. G.R. Burrus E.F. Busiek

W.M. Clark J.A. Cortner O.B. Crofford, Jr. D.L. Dolan J.A. Foley A.W. Graham, Jr. J.D. Gross W.H. Hall, Jr.

S.S. Haskell J.D. Hefner C.J. Hobdy G.R. Johnston D.A. Killen R.G. Long A.E. Lyons R.M. McKey, Jr.

J.S. McMurry C.K. Meador H.N. Meiers E.W. Moore R.B. Moore, Jr. C.H. Nicholson M.C. Peper P.P. Porch, Jr.

W. Puckett, III R.E. Ray E.M. Regen, Jr. V.H. Reynolds J.O. Rice R.S. Sanders M.H. Schwartz R.D. Sellers

C.H. Smith M.R. Stocking J.L. Story H.S. Street G.R. Swafford V.A. Utley J.R. Wilson W.B. Wilson

The class of 1955.

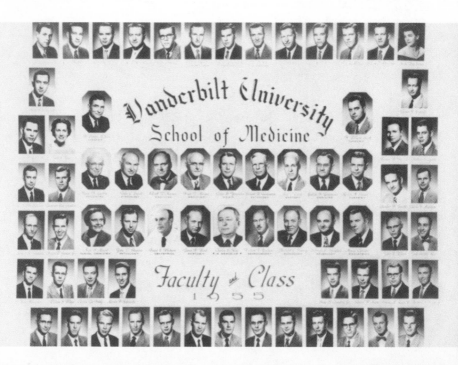

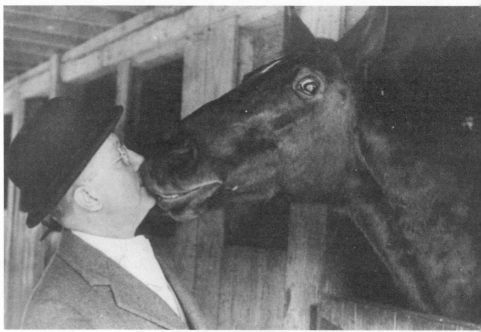

Top: The class of 1955. **Bottom:** *Dean John Youmans and one of his horses.*

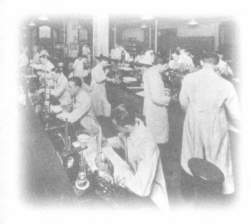

11

TOOLS OF
THE TRADE

2. Introduction to Clinical Medicine. — An integrated course given by members of the Departments of Biochemistry, Medicine, Radiology, and Surgery. Lectures, demonstrations, and practical experience are designed to introduce students to methods used in examining patients and to the interpretation of data so obtained. This course serves also as a transition from the courses in biochemistry, physiology, and pathology to their application in clinical medicine. The course consists of fourteen lectures or demonstrations and six hours of practical demonstrations, weekly, during the third trimester of the second year. Dr. Kampmeier and Dr. Hartman.

Each student is required to possess a standard, 4 objective microscope, equipped with a substage light. All students are required to provide themselves with hemocytometers, hemoglobinometers, and ophthalmoscopes before the beginning of the 2nd trimester of the 2nd year.

Catalogue for 1952–1953
School of Medicine
Vanderbilt University

AFTER CHRISTMAS BREAK OF THE SECOND YEAR, WE BEGAN the Introduction to Clinical Medicine course. The load was no lighter than the year before—we carried this course along with Pharmacology, Parasitology, Microbiology, and a new course called Clinical Pathology. But we also were beginning to move from a lab and lecture format to dealing with patients. In Introduction to Clinical Medicine, we would learn to take a medical history and perform a physical examination.

We could not have had a better teacher for the course. Dr. Rudolph Kampmeier literally wrote the book on the subject—*Physical Examination in Health and Disease*, the standard textbook then used across the nation by most medical schools.

After our first class session, where Dr. Kampmeier told us what to expect from the course and what he expected, we raced to the surgical supply store on the edge of the campus to buy the clinical instruments that would become a staple of our professional lives. I returned to my room and started opening the packages. Each instrument was wrapped in white tissue paper, and the excitement I felt in opening them was the same that I felt on Christmas mornings as a child. The consideration of new toys and new tools shares a distinct flavor—the anticipation of frequent usage. I arranged the instruments across the bed in rows and just sat there a bit, taking it all in. Then I began examining each instrument.

I took the ophthalmoscope apart several times, shined the little light, rotated the various lenses, and adjusted the diopter focusing device. What would I see *inside* eyes? Then I attached the otoscope and its earpieces. I removed the bulb to see how it worked and then selected several different sizes of earpieces. When and for what would I use each one?

I hung my new stethoscope around my neck and stood before the mirror. Though I had just turned twenty-one, I looked like a boy with a stethoscope around his neck.

I put the stethoscope on my bare chest and listened to the lubdub lubdub. What sense could I ever make out of these sounds? I knew of heart murmurs, but I had no idea how they sounded. I listened to my watch with the stethoscope, and then I whispered into the bell to hear the magnified tones of my voice. I picked up the red rubber reflex hammer and tapped on my knee until I evoked some semblance of a knee jerk.

Of all the items, the hemoglobinometer and blood cell counter set were my favorites. They came in a neat case, convenient to take to the wards. We would do all the hematology lab work on our patients with this small kit. I had no idea how the parts worked. There were several different shaped pipettes and a hand counter device. There were glass counting chambers with small etched lines for counting white and red cells and platelets. There was a device with a spring-loaded needle for puncturing fingers. We would use it over and over with only alcohol wipes in between. (Fears of blood-transmitted diseases were still in the future.) In a few months, I would know all about these instruments, be able to use them accurately, and measure all the components of blood on real patients. But for now I just sat there, fascinated. These were the tools of my profession. They were my future. For nearly an hour, I examined the pieces of my future, picking them up again and again, in a state more trance than waking . . . the future.

The next day we switched from the long white lab coats worn by freshmen and sophomores into the short white coats of the juniors and seniors. We had arrived. That first walk outside the medical school in my short white coat with my stethoscope sticking out of my pocket is still vivid in my memory. On days like that, the sun shines brighter and colors are more vivid. The trees were just coming out in their spectacular spring green. If sap can rise in a human being, the sap was rising that first day in short white coats as our group ambled toward the Phi Chi house for lunch.

After years of preparation, we were finally about to make contact with real live patients. But first we would exhaustively practice on the bodies of each other as we struggled to learn and internalize Kampmeier's teachings.

A medical history consists of four distinct elements. First, there is the chief complaint, then the story of the present illness, then the review of organ systems. Finally, there is the past history, which consists of the past medical, personal, social, and family history. We took histories on each other for several weeks. As none of our classmates had any interesting diseases in their past, we were soon bored with the nearly normal.

We described and observed only the "normal" for weeks. Dr. Kampmeier never let us use the terms "normal" or "negative" in our descriptions. Whatever the area of the body was, we had to write a description of what we saw, felt, heard, or even smelled—every sense except taste. "Inspection, palpation, and auscultation," he said over and over again and in that order. It was one of his several litanies. We habituated the sequence—same routine in the same order. LOOK! FEEL! LISTEN! "Look for what you are going to feel. Feel for what you are going to listen to. Listen to what you have seen and felt." Olfaction was not in the list, but he told stories of the characteristic smells of some diseases.

We wrote detailed descriptions in our weekly examinations of each other. For example, as I tried to describe the acneform rash of my partner, I might write, "The skin of the forehead is yellowish pink and clear of any visible lesions. There are red raised areas scattered around the edge of each side of the nose. These measure between two and four millimeters in diameter. Some have yellow white centers. Others are excoriated with small dark red centers." At this stage we could not use any medical terms. We had to describe as though we were lay people looking at another person in great detail, like Martians seeing Earthlings for the first time.

Even when we eventually began to see real patients, we continued to write detailed descriptions. We could never say a part was "normal" or within "normal limits." Kampmeier detested the term "negative." He argued that usage of these terms was earned by repeated careful observations of the normal. We would have no idea of what was normal or abnormal until we had seen patients for a long time. Besides, variations of normal are frequent, so we would have to slowly learn to make distinctions between these variations and the variations that come from disease. He preferred the terms "absent" or "present," so long as we specified what was or was not present. For example, we would write, "There was no redness and no swelling visible in any area of the neck."

Dr. Kampmeier read every write-up in detail and used red ink extensively. He was like a fine English teacher who spends time marking themes and pieces of creative writing, correcting here, adding there, or striking whole paragraphs. Our write-ups could easily go for twelve or fifteen pages. No matter how long, he read them, corrected them, and returned our write-ups by the next session.

We quickly learned that, for Kampmeier, there was no such thing as "no symptoms." There was merely a long list of absent symptoms. Instead of writing "no symptoms of the ear or nose or throat," or whatever area of the body was being explored, we had to write, "no ear pain, no tinnitus, no discharge from the external meatus, no pruritus, no decreased hearing noted," and so on, building an exhaustive list of what was *not* complained about. This approach ensured that I gradually built an internal catalogue of every imaginable symptom for each organ system. By course's end I could say them by rote, and eventually, if I left a symptom off my list, an automatic alarm would sound in my brain. This learning has lasted a lifetime, and has proved invaluable to proper treatment, especially when the diagnosis is unclear.

The necessity of inquiring about all symptoms was driven home early in the course. Ben (my partner and roommate at the Phi Chi house) and I were trying to take a history on one of our first real patients. The woman, in her sixties, was from one of the poorer counties surrounding Nashville—"country people," we called them. She looked like she had led a hard life. She had no teeth, though she did have snuff stains on her lower lip, and her feet looked like they had never seen shoes. She had never married, and lived with her sister and brother-in-law on a hillside farm, miles off of the nearest paved road. They had no electricity and no running water.

Ben and I put our clipboards with the printed long list of symptoms for each organ system between our legs; that way we could look down at the list of symptoms and refer to it, so we would not omit asking about each one. (It did not occur to me then that sitting before a patient with a clipboard between my knees was not the best way to establish rapport.)

There was nothing spontaneous about the woman. When asked why she was in the hospital, she replied, "'Cause the doctor told me to come here."

For well over an hour, we asked about this symptom and that symptom, all the way down from her head to her feet. When we had finished the list, I looked at Ben, and he looked at me. We had no clue as to what this woman had. To each symptom, she had answered, "Nope, ain't had none of that." In contrast to patients who have too many symptoms, this woman had none. We had no idea why she was in the hospital. Again we scanned the list of symptoms on the clipboards in our laps, and then Ben, out of nowhere, asked, "How much water do you drink?" We had inadvertently skipped "polydipsia" (excessive thirst).

"Oh, 'bout three gallons a day," the woman replied, in a bored voice with as much emotion as if she had told us the time of day.

Ben and I looked at each other. While we felt triumphant at having ferreted out the woman's condition, we had violated one of the basic rules of good history taking. Instead of asking the woman to tell us her story, we had jumped right to interrogation. We asked "yes" and "no" questions, and we got "yes" and "no" answers. She went on to explain that thirty years earlier a mule had kicked her in the head, knocking her down and out. Ever since then, she had to drink gallons of water a day to keep up with her thirst. Since she lived on a hill and the well was down in the hollow, every night she and her sister had to haul enough water up the hill for her to make it through the night. This had been going on for three decades. She would not even have been here now had her sister not fallen ill. The doctor treating her sibling had found out about the water drinking and sent her to Vanderbilt Hospital.

She had diabetes insipidus caused by the absence of anti-diuretic hormone. When the mule kicked her, the blow caused a severance of the stalk of the pituitary gland at the base of her brain. This stopped the secretion of anti-diuretic hormone, thus allowing the kidney to excrete excessive amounts of dilute urine. She had suffered from the condition for so long that she did not even see it as abnormal or unusual.

A few days later, we found by reading her chart that the woman had refused the daily injections that would have normalized her urine output and thirst. Apparently, when she refused the treatment, she had told the intern, "No thanks, I'd just as soon keep toting water."

In addition to learning the value of asking about every specific symptom, she embodied one of Kampmeier's most oft-repeated lessons: Patients will often tell you exactly what is wrong with them if you let them. We never gave the woman time to do that.

Kampmeier did more than lecture about subtle and effective history taking—he was himself somewhat of a legend. He had a long list of clinical triumphs to his credit, of which two in particular come to mind. The first occurred during teaching rounds in our senior year. Kampmeier was my attending physician. We were walking from room to room on the private wing. In addition to his teaching load, he had a busy private referral practice. We came to the adjoining rooms of an elderly couple. Both were missionaries from somewhere in Africa. They had lived in the jungles with the natives to escape capture by the German army, and thus managed to survive World War II. Both had aneurysms of the ascending thoracic aorta, one of the classic manifestations of tertiary syphilis.

Kampmeier was a world-renowned expert on syphilis. In addition to his textbook on physical diagnosis, he had written the leading text on syphilis, *Essentials of Syphilology*. Sir William Osler said, "To know syphilis in all its manifestations is to know medicine." Kampmeier *knew* syphilis.

We stood in the hallway and spoke in hushed tones, out of hearing of the patients. One of our classmates presented the history, obviously proud to include many details he thought would please Kampmeier. When he finished, Kampmeier asked, "Now what about the primary lesion . . . the chancre?"

The student blushed and responded that he had been too embarrassed to ask such a question of missionaries, especially elderly ones. Kampmeier instructed us to wait outside the room. He entered the man's room. Minutes later, Kampmeier appeared back in the hall. He had a habit of pursing his lips into a small snout and moving the snout about, reminiscent of a wise rabbit. His neatly trimmed mustache wiggled back and forth at the end of his snout. He pursed his lips as a kind of punctuation to indicate the end of a point he was making.

"The old gentlemen tells me that . . . regrettably, one day . . . he wandered off into the jungle . . . with a young native girl . . . that would be over twenty years ago . . . became overwhelmed with lust . . . had sexual intercourse. Says it was his only transgression. A few days later he noted a small sore . . . on the side of his penis . . . junction of the glans just below the meatus, to be exact . . . thought nothing of it at the time." Each brief phrase was punctuated by a pursing of his lips. All very matter of fact. "Skipped the secondary phase, not uncommon . . . very important to get the history of the primary. Can't be sure without the chancre history. Takes a bit of prompting . . . careful questioning."

In his lectures, Kampmeier had driven home time and again that syphilis was no respecter of age, sex, education, or position in life. He had seen it in the lowly and the high. No one and no profession or level of education was granted immunity. Seeing two elderly missionaries with tertiary syphilis of the aorta cemented that point in my mind.

The episode taught me more than just another lesson about Kampmeier's skill. It was a lesson in the role discretion should play in diagnosis. My classmate had been too restrained in his history taking, allowing embarrassment to interfere with the diagnosis. But once the true story was uncovered, there was an obligation *not* to tell more than was one's concern.

In this case, Kampmeier assured the man that he would not tell the wife about her husband's transgression. Both were told of the nature of their illness, and both were treated for third stage syphilis, but Kampmeier said it was up to the man, not him, to tell or not tell the wife the whole story. Kampmeier would make no judgment about the issue, considering it purely a matter between the man and his wife. The wife knew what she had but had no idea how she had gotten it. It was not our duty as physicians to intrude where we were neither needed nor welcomed. Kampmeier believed that medicine is amoral, not immoral, but amoral. As doctors, we were not to pass judgment on anyone's morals. We were to treat murderers with the same attention as anyone else—to comfort and heal, not to judge behavior.

The other case that demonstrated Kampmeier's impressive ability to draw out the truth of a medical history involved a young man who had been repeatedly admitted to the hospital with a curious set of findings. Each time he was admitted with high fever and palpable air under the skin of his upper body—subcutaneous emphysema. He would come into the hospital, get cultured, and be started on streptomycin and penicillin, recover, and go home only to be readmitted in a few months with the same findings. No one had the slightest clue as to the cause of this strange syndrome.

On one admission he was presented at the weekly medical grand rounds. This was the event of the week, and the entire third and fourth year classes attended along with most of the clinical faculty. One of the attendings led the discussion. He discussed every conceivable gas-forming bacillus and indulged in a wide swathe of speculation as to what organism could do such things, even though no case of infected spontaneous subcutaneous emphysema could be found in the literature. All matter of imaginative fistulae between lung and skin, esophagus and skin, pharynx and skin, and others were presented as possibilities. None was ever found. Most concluded that the young man had his own unique disease, whatever it was. The case history was famous. All residents eagerly anticipated the next admission, waiting to get their shot at solving the puzzle.

And the readmissions continued, each time as puzzling as the last. Finally, someone thought to ask Kampmeier to see the patient. Kampmeier chose to see the patient late one evening, after all the visitors had gone home. After speaking to the man alone, Kampmeier emerged, answer in hand. The young man lived in the country, as did his girlfriend. The man's father ran a gas station between the two houses. The couple would meet frequently at night in the back of the closed gas station and have sexual intercourse, but not the usual kind. His girlfriend had strange ideas about sex.

Occasionally, she insisted on biting a small hole in the skin of his upper arm. She would then insert a football air needle into the hole in the skin and pump in air with a bicycle pump. The young man said she liked the crunchy feel of the air under the skin. Most times it caused no trouble. Whenever he got a fever, he knew to go immediately to the hospital. The mystery was solved, and Kampmeier's stock went even higher. If you can get a history like that, you can get a history from anybody.

Kampmeier saw disease as a unique interaction between a person, the people around him, and the setting or environment in which he lives—including the food eaten, the air breathed, and the bacteria, viruses, and parasites surrounding him. For him, the story of the disease was the story of the person. He would often say, "What is the man's story? Don't get lost in the details of all the disease names. Tell me the story of his illness."

He preferred to go back to the beginning of the illness, to a time when the person was last feeling completely well and healthy and start there. I often used that later in my practice.

Kampmeier's rounds in the clinic or on the wards demonstrated his mastery of the diagnostic process. We presented the cases to him. He only wanted the history, and he spent a lot of time on the details of it. He wanted to know everything you could possibly know about a pain. Where was it? Did it radiate or move? Did the man point at it with one finger, or did he use his whole hand? Did he use the back of his hand or the palm of his hand when he pointed to the pain? Was his hand made into a fist, or was his hand open when he pointed at the site? Did he smile or frown when he talked about the pain? What time of day did the pain occur, at night, during the day, before or after meals, and if so, how long after meals? How long did the pain last? What was the "shape" of the pain? Did it come on abruptly or slowly? Did the pain wobble up and down in intensity, or was it constant? He could go on with questions about pain for what seemed like forever, especially if you were presenting or if you did not know the answers about your patient.

Kampmeier gave us a lot of useful pearls about taking histories. One of the best was his admonition to repeat the description of the symptom back to the patient. "If you are on target with your description, the patient will nod agreement. You will see it in their eyes. They know and you know that you understand how they feel. You have described it back to them. Only then can you know what that symptom really feels like to your patient." It is a powerful method, and one I used for the rest of my life in practice.

Sometimes in presentations, he would summarize what he had learned from the history. He would then tell us in detail what the physical exam would or would not show. Most of the time the physical exam would add little or no new information. It might only confirm what the history told him, but by no means did he advocate a sloppy or casual exam. He only made the point that the physical exam was weak compared to the history. He used the physical exam to confirm or refute the diagnostic possibilities from the history and also to look for signs of disease that were not yet symptomatic. After the physical, he then told us what the lab work would show or not show. He thought of lab work as only confirmatory. He saw lab work as an extension of the physical exam, and had the opinion that tests should only be ordered in response to findings from the history or physical exam. One segment of the diagnostic process led to the next segment in a logical order. History begat the physical exam begat the lab work, and so on, in an iterative fashion.

When I think back to the beginning of that semester, I still recall the excitement I felt that day in the Phi Chi house, as I stood in my room looking at all those new instruments. Those gleaming instruments carried so much promise. And by the end of Kampmeier's course, I had indeed explored and used them and come to understand the extent to which such instruments advanced and enabled the more adept practice of medicine. But by then, Kampmeier's methods had impressed upon me how limited any medical instrument is. No stethoscope can detect such emotions as shame or embarrassment, and no ophthalmoscope can tell what a patient has seen and done. Only the patient can tell the doctor these things. Fortunately, if trained and honed, we all have the very tool needed to work in these areas where others fall short—the human mind.

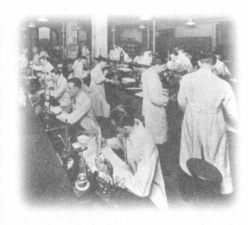

12

THE
PERFECT SMEAR

Clinical Pathology. — A series of lectures and laboratory exercises in the micro-
scopic and chemical methods in the diagnosis of disease. Students are trained in
the technique of examining urine, blood, sputum, gastric contents, feces, and
"puncture fluids." The interpretation of laboratory data is discussed. Eight hours
a week during the 3rd trimester of the second year. Dr. Hartman.

Catalogue for 1952–1953
School of Medicine
Vanderbilt University

IF ANYONE WONDERS WHY HEALTH CARE COSTS HAVE RISEN,
one need only look at the status of medical testing in university hospitals
prior to the introduction of Medicare coverage in 1966. Before
Medicare, all lab work was done by medical students at no charge. It
was scut work, and there was plenty of it. While there was a nominal
charge for blood chemistries and X-rays, all other tests were free.
Hospital workers were specifically excluded from the minimum
wage law, and many worked for a dollar an hour or less. The entire
enterprise was low tech and low cost. In the place of sophisticated
equipment and testing, clinical reasoning reigned supreme. The cost
of medical care was mostly paid by cash or written off as charity. There
was little or no health insurance. Patients were very careful about
having tests even when their physician had ordered them. In the clinic,
they often refused to have tests done if they could not afford them. The

lack of funds made it imperative for doctors to have a sharpened clinical acumen and to avoid unnecessary testing, and for medical students to quickly develop these skills. But no matter how sharp the doctor, sloppy lab work could slow down or even derail a diagnosis. It was the responsibility of Dr. Robert Hartman to ensure that we performed all lab work, no matter how routine, with the skill and attention that guaranteed the results would be the boon to diagnosis intended.

We met Dr. Hartman just after the Christmas break of our second year. He taught Clinical Pathology, a subsection of Dr. Rudolph Kampmeier's Introduction to Clinical Medicine. In this course we would be taught all the laboratory methods we would use in actually doing a variety of blood counts, urinalyses, spinal fluid analyses, stool examinations, and other lab work on the patients we would see in the coming junior year. The only tests medical students did not do were blood chemistries, which were done in a separate lab.

While we would work with a variety of bodily fluids and substances, it is blood with which I associate the course and Dr. Hartman. To some degree this is simply due to quantity. Medical students drew all the blood for testing for the entire hospital and all of the clinics, and blood would be the principal medium in which we worked. But beyond the practical and mundane, there was something more. Here was a man with a name the slightest degree removed from "Heart Man" teaching a course in blood. And he began with a splash.

In one of his first lectures, Hartman kept us waiting. Next to the podium where he usually spoke, there was a clean white bed sheet draped over a large wooden stand. After all of the class had arrived and had a few minutes to settle in and start wondering about what purpose the sheet served, Hartman entered quickly, followed by two women. Though we would come to know them as Dorothy and Susan, the two technicians who assisted in the course looked at the moment for all the world like two lovely female assistants on stage to aid their boss—the magician—about to perform some astounding feat. The women quickly unfurled another sheet, obstructing our view of the Great Hartman-dini. Moments later, the sheet was whipped aside, revealing Hartman standing in front of a blood-soaked bed sheet. Susan and Dorothy, obviously aware of how all of this looked, stepped to each side, bowed, and extended their hands toward Hartman. For his own part, Hartman seemed still taken by the act he had performed behind the sheet. He raised both arms high in the air and stepped around in small circles.

After a few circuits, he paused and spoke. "Now, let's have estimates of the amount of blood I just threw on the sheet," he announced in a loud voice. When he spoke, the illusion of Hartman as master magician was somewhat shaken. He lacked a voice that commanded a stage. His voice always sounded like he needed to clear his throat, and when he raised the volume it sounded like he was gargling.

Dorothy went to the blackboard and began to line off several columns. Hartman called out the names of the students in the first row, then the next row, until everyone had made an estimate. (One of Hartman's first acts of minor magic was learning all of our names by the end of the first week.) Our guesses ranged from 50 cc's to 300 cc's with an average of about 200 cc's. The sheet looked like it had been dipped in blood, and I would have guessed a quart of blood if others had not guessed so low.

Hartman smiled widely, almost giggling, as he ran off the numbers in the hand-cranked adding machine—the closest equivalent to a calculator the 1950s had to offer—he had brought to class.

"Of course, I could calculate the mean and standard deviation of the mean, but I won't do that. Anyone know why?" He paused, glanced back over his shoulder with pride, but did not wait for the answer. "Well, we all know that since we have the universe of answers and not simply a sample of the universe, that we do not need to make any calculation of variance. We can see the variance right there on the blackboard."

Then, with our interest peaked and anticipation building, Hartman wandered off for several minutes into a lengthy presentation about statistics and the detailed methods of calculations. When he lapsed into these frequent digressions, his voice shifted to a softer and lower pitch. His facial expression lost its intensity. If his voice detracted from his attempts at showmanship, his digressions into arcane methodologies and statistical formulas derailed them completely. It was as if two distinct personalities battled for control. Instead of Jekyll and Hyde, there was a less dramatic but still incongruous conflict between Academic Researcher and Master Showman, and the latter never held the stage for long. One moment, Hartman was an amateurish but enthusiastic magician eager to astound, then—poof!—he would transform into the preoccupied academic researcher. Sometimes he seemed aware of a digression, and he would shake his head and blink his eyes as if to force himself out of it. At other times he would come out of them and look vacant for a few moments, much like the post-ictal state of confusion after grand mal seizures. As befits a good digression, what he said about statistics this day had nothing to do with the subject at hand—estimating blood loss.

So we sat there, the expertly built-up anticipation draining away, and—poof!—the showman reasserted himself. Hartman reached into his pocket and, with an exaggerated flourish, produced a small vial of blood. Holding it high so everyone could see it, he announced in a gargle, "The actual amount of blood was 10 cc's, as in this vial." He turned to one of his assistants. "Susan, please put up a clean sheet for my next demonstration." As the new sheet was prepared, Hartman held the small vial high above his head and slowly walked down the first row of seats before returning to the sheet.

Stepping back, he took the vial of blood and lunged toward the sheet, flinging the blood toward the clean sheet. Blood went all over it. The sheet was drenched. Ten cc's splashed like a quart. Hartman then stepped toward the open window and tossed the empty vial out of the window onto the courtyard below. His improbable gesture had the celebratory flair of the flinging of a champagne glass into the fireplace after the last toast of the evening.

Hartman turned to the class, obviously pleased. "Never let it be said that you did not learn the true problem of estimating blood loss. Gentlemen, it cannot be done from observation alone. You must measure it. In the case of clothing or bedclothes or even operative lap sheets, blood loss cannot be estimated. Surgeons cannot do it, nor can patients." He then went into a long description of weighing, then drying, then reweighing the bloody cloths or sponges. From the differences in weight, one could exactly calculate the amount of blood. The method was impractical, but it illustrated Hartman's zeal for accuracy.

It was an important lesson. While we would learn to hone and rely upon our eyes and judgment, there was the danger we would do so to the extent that we trusted eye and judgment too much. Hartman's presentation reinforced for us the importance of the very techniques we were in the class to learn.

While Hartman's act on stage with the sheets was flamboyant, he demanded each of us perform our own feat with blood, even making it a requirement for passing his course. To pass, each of us was required to produce one perfect blood smear. Using two small glass cover slips, we put a drop of blood on one glass slip, dropped a second glass slip onto the blood and then quickly pulled the glass slips apart, leaving a fine smear of blood on both slips. We then stained the two smears. Hartman detested the method of a slide being pulled against another slide, the one used by most people. He spoke with passion and some animation about the errors that the old two-slide method could produce. It was a subject that caused him to raise his voice to full gargle as he held forth about the idiocy of using a crude slide to make something as important as a blood smear.

Hartman was exacting and precise in his definitions of the perfect blood smear. The perfect slide would have no red blood cell in the entire smear touching another cell. None. If he found any cells touching, he rejected the slide. The distance between any two cells could not exceed the diameter of two red blood cells. Whenever we thought we had a perfect smear, we would call him over to our microscope and have him peer at the slide and make his pronouncement. He would straddle the lab stool, slide his glasses onto his head, and look into the scope. He then quickly moved the slide around a bit, and most of the time, look up and tell us why the slide was imperfect. Sometimes it would only be a few cells barely touching or a spot where the blood thinned out on the edges. Each time he rejected what I hoped was a perfect smear, I would feel a sickening sensation in my stomach. I knew I would pull many more before any came close to being perfect.

At any spare moment, often at night, we sat at the long black benches of the student lab. At first we used each other's stuck fingers, but that slowed us down too much. We soon learned to stick our own fingers. We sat there night after night at the end of our studies, sticking our fingers with a sharp needle, letting the blood drip, and then pulling slide after slide of our own blood. After we had a dozen or more, we then stained the best blood smears with Wright's stain.

And Hartman not only demanded the perfect smear; he also expected the perfect stain, with just the correct amount of blue and pink and no precipitate of stain showing. It was frustrating to pull a perfect slide but then mess it up with the staining process. I don't know how many slides it took to get what would pass as perfect, but it must have been hundreds. Granted, this process taught us how to pull slides quickly and properly, and we would use that skill over and over in the following years of medical school and in internship. But it seemed teaching overkill. We grumbled and railed, away from faculty ears, about mind-numbing repetition and the obsessive-compulsive nitpicking of it all.

Eventually, all of us did pull a perfect slide, and despite all of our complaints, Hartman taught us there is a correct and an incorrect method to do anything. More importantly, in a course that began with a splash and ended in a smear, we learned about the essence of perfection, a lesson that sank in slowly but went deep. When perfection is achieved, it is earned. But like those who salute the journey over the destination, it is the pursuit of perfection as much as its attainment that yields the most valuable dividends for the student and, later, the doctor. By learning *how* to strive for perfection in the smallest of things, we learned why such striving matters.

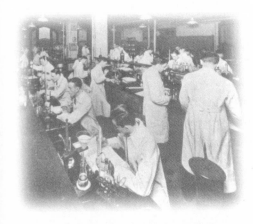

13

A SOLO FLIGHT
INTO A HISTORY

*230. Medicine. Clinical Lectures and Demonstrations. Patients are presented by
the students to whom they are assigned.*

Catalogue for 1952–1953, page 80
School of Medicine
Vanderbilt University

THE CLINICAL COURSES WITH KAMPMEIER AND HARTMAN
were in the final month of the second year. We would soon be on the
wards and in the clinical clerkships. The clerkships consisted of three-
month rotations in the major clinical fields of medicine and surgery.
Pediatrics and obstetrics had six weeks for each. Everything else was
considered a subspecialty and would be covered by clinic rotations in
the senior year. We were in the final stages of our preparation to work
directly with patients and be a part of the team of interns and assistant
residents who actually cared for the patients.

In this final month of the course, we worked alone for the first time
with one patient at a time. I was in the very awkward phase of history
taking and still had to keep my history outline and list of symptoms on
a clipboard in my lap. I came to think that taking a history was literally
just that. I would ask questions about symptoms, and the patient would
answer. By the time I finished, I would have a list of all of his symptoms, dates, and names of previous diseases, operations, and present
medicines. I would also know what diseases his father and mother had,

and I would know something about the social history. The patient was there to answer my questions. That's what I thought, until I encountered Lemuel Harrison on my solo flight into history taking.

Mr. Lemuel Harrison was a sixty-nine-year-old farmer from Cheatham County, one of five counties ringing Nashville. These counties were called rim counties because of their location around the city, and because they formed a high rim of sand and limestone around the deep basin where Nashville sat. Geologically, all of this was the residual runoff from millions of years of erosion from the worn-down Appalachian Mountains to the east. Mr. Harrison lived in the poorest of the rim counties, where the soil was so poor the only crop was corn, and the only cash came from bootleg corn whiskey.

Mr. Harrison was on 3300, the all-male, sixteen-bed surgical ward. He was in the third bed on the left, with a commanding view of the entire ward. Each bed had a curtain hung from a rail that could be pulled around to create a modicum of privacy. I quickly found that the curtain did not block out any sound.

He was propped up on pillows when I walked to the bedside. About seven or eight men in robes and pajamas moved back, sliding their chairs out of the way as I approached. The great sultan was dismissing his court.

"Well, better hold it for now, boys. Got me a new doctor," Mr. Harrison announced in an unusually loud voice. I had not yet learned that he was partially deaf.

"You one of them learning doctors, ain't you?" Mr. Harrison asked. He slid his legs off of the edge of the bed, rose from his array of pillows, and brushed at his hair with his hand. "Like you learning how to doctor, ain't you?" That brought a few giggles from his tribe.

"Yes sir, I am," I said. I pulled the curtain around his bed and sat on the chair directly in front of him. He sat higher than me and cast a glance to both sides. In hindsight, I realized he was checking for his audience. Looking back on it now, I realize my big mistake was sitting lower than Mr. Harrison. I gave up whatever small advantage I had right away by sitting beneath him.

"Well, just shoot. Ax me any question you want," he said, sticking his arm straight up into the air to adjust the sleeves of his bathrobe.

"Well, what brought you to the hospital?" I asked, thinking I would let him tell his story and ramble a bit. I was not going to make the mistake we did with the woman who drank three gallons of water a day.

"What'd you say?" he answered. I had to learn to speak in a very loud voice, or I had to repeat everything. I suspected he still made me repeat the questions whenever he had a particularly good response. I repeated my question, inquiring about what brought him into the hospital.

"Hit was a '38 Ford," Mr. Harrison answered, chuckling to himself. Outside the thin curtain I could hear a few giggles, then chairs scraping, as a small audience regathered outside the curtain. The tribes were coming into session.

I learned right then and there never to phrase that question that way. I would learn a lot of things not to do before I finished the history of Mr. Harrison that day.

"I didn't mean what car brought you. What medical problem made you come?" I asked. I could feel my face redden. I felt a sinking feeling, realizing I was in for a tough time.

"Well, just to get right down to it. I can't pee like I used to." More giggles and some mumbling from outside the curtain.

I glanced at my list of questions, still not automatic in my questioning. "Do you mean your stream has decreased?" I asked.

"Why hell, yes. Use to be able to knock a hole in a collard leaf from twenty feet." He paused to wait out the guffaws and thigh slapping from outside the curtain. "Tell 'em, Lem," I heard one of them call out. His timing was perfect.

"Now I couldn't knock a hole in a wet paper napkin." The audience grew larger, I could tell from the scraping of more chairs. No one wanted to miss this. Now there were little echoes of responses from the gathered group. "Tell 'em, old man." More giggles and a few loud laughs.

"Matter of fact, my pecker won't do a lot of things it used to." Mr. Harrison just threw that in. By this time he had a full house outside the curtain.

I struggled through a long rambling story of his life on the farm, his three wives and thirteen children, the Great Depression, his part in World War I, and his sons' parts in World War II. He claimed to personally know Sergeant Alvin York, the legendary war hero from Tennessee. He said he grew up in the valley next to him up near Jamestown in Fentress County, and later moved to Cheatham County when he got married to the first wife. Each story brought more and more laughter. Mr. Harrison was completely in charge, and I was struggling to get through all the questions I was supposed to ask. I had gone too far in letting the patient tell his story.

One phase of the history taking is called the review of systems, where symptoms for each organ are explored systematically. This starts with the head and progresses through the heart, lungs, GI tract, and kidneys on down to the feet and legs. I had slowly wound my way down to the GI tract and was checking out his bowel habits.

"How are your bowel habits?" I asked.

"What'd you say?" he asked.

"Your bowel habits. Your stools. How are they?" I raised my voice a good bit.

"Can't hear you," he said, leaning toward me with his head tilted to one ear. I knew somehow in the deep part of my brain that I was being set up.

"BOWEL HABITS. YOUR STOOLS. CAN YOU GO TO THE TOILET?" I was just under yelling.

"Oh, I got you. Hell yes, take a dump every day of my life." That brought down the house. By this time, he must have had the entire ward and all the visitors outside the curtain. I had just about given up any semblance of being professional. I was beginning to enjoy the session, and didn't mind feeding him straight lines.

I had reviewed all the organ systems for symptoms and was now attempting to get his "social history."

"What other jobs have you had other than farming?"

"Sho'. Got it. I makes corn licker."

"How do you do it?" I asked. I was fascinated.

"Well, I puts in corn and barley, and lots of sugar and water. Makes a mash. Put all that in a big wooden tub. Takes some time to work, you know, ferment. Course I crank it up some. Yup, I crank it up." He paused, waiting. I took the bait.

"Crank it up, what's that?" I asked.

"Well, I do it special," he answered. "I put in a shovel or two of horse manure."

"Horse what?" I asked, not believing what he just said.

"HORSE SHIT, SONNY, HORSE SHIT." The ward erupted in laughter. Now there were shouts, everyone joined in. I felt like I was at a wrestling match with the crowd gone wild. "Tell 'em old man." "Go to it!" "That's some real whiskey." "Man, I ain't coming near your house!" "Whoever heard of horse shit whiskey?" Finally the crowd settled back down.

"Why do you put horse manure in your mash?" I asked.

"Gives the whiskey a special bite."

I went by to see Mr. Harrison every day and chatted with him. He had his prostate operated on and stayed in the hospital for nearly two weeks. He told me stories of growing up in the Tennessee mountains, of hunting wild turkeys, of square dancing, of courting his first wife. He had shot wild bears and, in the early days, saw wolves still in the region. His grandfather had settled in the mountains, moving from the Carolinas, and had known Indians who still lived in the area.

Mr. Harrison taught me a lot about history taking. I would slowly learn how to be directive, yet leave room for patients to move freely when necessary into their own stories. I would find that the real important information came when the patient was allowed to talk, and that "yes" and "no" questions brought only "yes" and "no" responses. It is a fine line to keep the history flowing, and yet cover all that is needed to gather the necessary information. In later years, I would find that some histories take weeks or months to take. Some take years to fill out the full narrative of a person's life and its relationship to his health and illnesses. Illness is largely a personal narrative, and to miss the full narrative is to miss so much about understanding disease in a given individual. I learned the truth of the old saw that it is as important to know the patient with the disease as it is to know the disease. Some people do quite well with diseases that incapacitate others.

It was necessary for us to learn to do a full history in one setting, but that process gave an artificial compression of what it would be like in practice to see patients over long periods of time. Only then would I realize how slowly some people's stories unfold and how impossible it is to gather any more than a meager picture of a life in less than an hour.

Mr. Harrison had a wonderful life, and he shared it with me and taught me much about people. I will always be grateful to him. All of my patients were my teachers. He was one of my best.

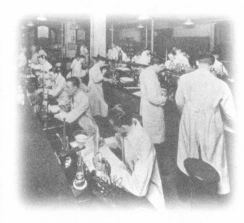

14

THE
SILVER
PHANTOM

Although there is no scheduled time for extracurricular activities, I suggest periodic breaks from your study routines as a way of refreshing your minds.

Remarks from the Dean
Fall 1951

LATE ONE EVENING CLOSE TO MIDNIGHT, TOWARD THE end of the second year, I found Oscar sitting in the living room of the Phi Chi house. He was holding a large can of paint by the handle.

"Look at what I found in the hall closet," he said.

It was a gallon of metallic silver paint and several paint brushes. New and unopened. We both stared at the can.

"Let's paint the doorknobs silver," I blurted out.

"Exactly what I was thinking," Oscar said. "And then say nothing. Wait until someone spots it."

We laid out our plan. We would paint just a few doorknobs silver and wait. We agreed to deny any part in it and create a mystery. That night we painted three doorknobs and the frame of one of the pictures a bright metallic silver. Then we hid the paint.

No one noticed over the next two days. It took all of our willpower to say nothing. Oscar and I agreed to meet again late at night when everyone was in bed and paint some more. The next night we painted all the knobs in the living room and the keyholes, too. Then we went on a spree and painted the rim of the television set, all the picture frames in the hallway downstairs, and the front doorknob and doorknocker.

The next night was Friday with all its ceremony, Oscar's latest letter from his mother, and the bestowing of the Horny Steer Award for the horniest student of the week. Someone had found a huge set of Texas Longhorn horns, so each week they were awarded to whoever could come up with the most absurd story about a classmate and some girl. Most of the stories were concocted, more fantasy than reality. Wally was telling us about Dr. Scott, the new chairman of surgery, and the terrors of the operating room. Someone mentioned the silver doorknobs. Someone else said the TV set was silver. With that, the dinner table emptied. We rushed upstairs to find out what else was silver.

We stood in the living room, looking at Oscar's and my handiwork. Wally yelled, "Look, they painted the picture frames." Jean said, "Check out the keyholes . . . all silver. What the hell is going on?"

The crowd was rushing about hunting for more silver objects. Within minutes everything we had painted had been found. Oscar and I rushed around looking like everyone else, calling out one or two things the others had missed. It was difficult to contain ourselves and not laugh. The response exceeded our wildest imagination. The place went berserk.

Wally named it. "It's the Silver Phantom. Somebody is painting this house silver. It's got to be one of those AKKs."

The AKK house, the other medical fraternity, was next door across a vacant lot. We moved freely back and forth between the two houses, and paid little or no attention to who belonged to which. The only time we paid any attention was on Saturday nights, when we played date hunting and capture between the two houses, but that is another long story.

For days the AKKs remained the number-one suspects. Oscar and I egged on those suspicions. Oscar insisted we wait to do any more painting. I wanted to go at it again the first night the painting was discovered. We waited. The tension rose. Every night at supper, it was the main topic of discussion. Who was the Silver Phantom? Everyone was looking for newly painted objects.

After several days, Oscar and I laid plans for the next painting attack. We had hidden the paint in a corner under the house so no one could find it. We decided to come in early from studying when no one was in the house, do our painting, then go back to the hospital and walk back to the house with the late crowd. That night, we painted just about everything in sight. We did the frame of the door to the living room, the light fixture in the ceiling, the window locks in the living room, the mullions in the front windows, the metal screen in the fireplace, and all the remaining doorknobs on the first floor. We were hard at it when Wally walked in.

"Well, I'll be damned. I can't believe it. You two." Wally sat in the chair, shook his head and laughed.

"OK, OK, you found us. Shut up and join us," Oscar quickly responded, "but keep your mouth shut. No blabbing." Oscar detested any kind of blabbering and predicted later that Wally would be unable to keep his mouth shut. "There's no way he can keep a secret."

Wally agreed and jumped right in, painting furiously. Laughing—painting—laughing—painting. He painted some of the spindles of the staircase to the upstairs. We cleaned up and rushed to the hospital just in time to walk back to the house with the study crowd. They went wild when they saw the fresh paint.

Wally went nuts along with the rest of the group. Wally was loudest of all, threatening the worst sort of things to whoever was the Silver Phantom. All kinds of dire threats were made. One member of the group wanted to call the police. We squelched that idea quickly. We sat around the living room trying to figure out how to find the Silver Phantom. Finally, everyone gave up and went to bed.

It took all of our powers to keep Wally from blabbing. We knew that he wanted to confess so he would get credit for being the phantom. Every night at supper we had to make faces at him to keep him quiet whenever the subject of the silver paint came up.

Everyone was so vigilant, we could not paint again. We had all agreed that we would rotate someone staying in the house to study so we could catch the phantom. We dared not paint when it was our turn to stay in the house since that would have been a dead giveaway.

Just as Oscar predicted, Wally could not stand the suspense. One Friday night he stood up and confessed, throwing Oscar and me in for good measure. The group erupted. They started yelling and throwing food and water at us, laughing and yelling. Then somebody yelled, "Let's hose 'em!" With that, they grabbed Wally, while Oscar and I ran for the steps. We made it to the front yard, only to be caught, held, and hosed down with icy water. The group, now drenched and shivering in the cold, doubled up with laughter, ambled back into the living room, and collapsed into the chairs. Everyone took turns telling who they thought the Silver Phantom was. We laughed until we couldn't laugh any more. Oscar, in his usual excessive detail, told his version of what we did. Then I told mine. Wally told his version, constantly interrupted and corrected by Oscar. Each story brought more laughing. Finally, we went to bed exhausted but also exhilarated. I could hear bursts of laughter and giggling from the other rooms as everyone told and retold stories of the Silver Phantom. The house gradually settled down and quieted for the night.

The Silver Phantom was gone, but not forgotten. There were just not many limits on what deprived medical students would do for entertainment.

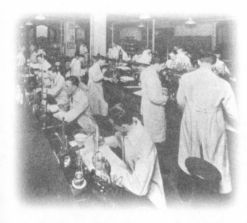

15

Surgeons
are Born,
Not Made

5. Surgical Ward. — For one trimester, one third of the third year students serve daily as assistants in the surgical wards of the Vanderbilt University Hospital. The students, under the direction of the staff, make records of the histories, physical examinations, and the usual laboratory tests. Ward rounds are made daily by various members of the surgical staff at which time surgical conditions are discussed with the students. The students may be present in the operating rooms at such times as their required work permits. When possible the student is permitted to assist in a surgical operation which is performed upon a patient assigned to him in the ward. Approximately twenty hours a week during one trimester of the third year.

Catalogue for 1953–1954
School of Medicine
Vanderbilt University

MY FIRST CLINICAL ROTATION OF THE THIRD YEAR WAS ON the surgical wards. There were two aspects to surgery I could not learn to accept—operating rooms and surgeons.

My first encounter set the tone. I was going to the fourth floor of the hospital, when the elevator stopped at the third floor. When the door opened, there stood a gnome in a long white coat. The elderly man was snarling at me. His long white coat nearly touched the floor, since he was barely over five feet tall.

"Get off this elevator," he said in a whining high-pitched voice. The locked psychiatric ward was just around the corner. I thought maybe one of the patients had escaped, disguised as a doctor. I backed further into the elevator.

"Get off. Now. Get off this elevator." He was hissing as he coiled into an even shorter height. I thought for a moment he was going to strike at me.

I didn't know what to do. I had noticed he had a stethoscope in his coat pocket. We stood there for a few seconds, staring at each other.

"Get off. Medical students don't ride elevators. Get off now." He was adamant.

As I slid by him on my way out, he said again, "Medical students don't ride elevators. Don't let me catch you again. Where do you think you got the time to spend lolly-gagging on some elevator? Medical students use the stairs."

I stood in the hallway wondering who and what that was all about. One of the medical residents wandered by, so I told him what had happened and described the man. He told me that must have been Dr. Barney Brooks, the retired chairman of surgery. To my great relief, it was the only time that I ever saw Dr. Brooks.

Barney Brooks was a legend of the school. He had been chairman of surgery for more than two decades, and had terrorized medical students and residents for all of that time. He had retired as chairman the year before.

There was an old story that was told over and over. Dr. Brooks was at the bottom of the pit in the amphitheater, conducting one of his teaching sessions. They always brought in the patient in a bed. Dr. Brooks was on one side, and the medical student was on the other side of the bed. The man had a duodenal ulcer and was being prepared for a gastric resection, the usual operation for intractable duodenal ulcers in those days. Dr. Brooks was discussing diet therapy, and he asked the student what he would feed the patient.

The medical student, already terror-struck, froze.

Dr. Brooks yelled in his high-pitched voice, "Well. What would you feed this patient?"

The student hesitated, paralyzed with fear.

Dr. Brooks yelled, "Well?"

Still in terror, he bumbled out, "mashed potatoes." Where that came from, no one knew.

Brooks wheeled around and yelled, "Mashed potatoes? MASHED POTATOES?"

The medical student fainted and fell to the floor. Brooks was about to continue his discussion when the medical student pulled himself up by the side rails on the bed. Brooks wheeled toward him again, "MASHED POTATOES. IS THAT ALL YOU CAN SAY?"

The story goes that the student fainted again. After my encounter on the elevator, I had no doubt about the truth of any story about Dr. Brooks.

There was one other encounter with a surgeon that removed any doubt about surgery as a career choice. I had been assigned to an orthopedic patient. The man, in his late fifties, had a fracture of the femur that required an open reduction. As the medical student, it was my job to take the initial history, do the physical examination, and perform all the routine lab work.

It was to be my first scrub on a real case. We had practiced scrubbing as part of the Introduction to Clinical Medicine course. We put black soot on our hands and then, blindfolded, we scrubbed for the required ten minutes. When the blindfolds were removed, we were startled to find out how much black material was still in between our fingers and under our nails. It was a great way to teach how thoroughly you must scrub to cleanse every part of the hand. We soon became quite good at it.

The official surgical scrub was ten minutes, using soap and a stiff hand brush. First we scrubbed from the elbow down the forearm to the wrist, then palms, and then the fingers and hands. When we got to the fingers, we systematically started on one finger (top, bottom, sides, and back) and slowly worked our way through all ten fingers. Then we put particular attention on the nails, being sure the bristles got underneath the nails. The webbing between the fingers, we had learned, was especially difficult to scrub clean, so we paid attention to those areas also.

When we finished, we rinsed from our hands down to our elbows, being careful to keep our hands in the air above the level of the elbows. This allowed the rinse water to run off our elbows and not back onto our hands.

The orthopedic surgeon, the resident, and the intern were already gowned and beginning the operation when I finished my scrub. I leaned against the swinging door with my back, being extra careful not to touch anything with my arms or hands. Now I was in the operating room. The surgeon spun around, looked at me and said, "Look out! You touched the I.V. pole. Get back in there and do a full ten minute re-scrub."

Just as I started to protest, the assistant resident turned and demanded, "Listen, snot, get in there and scrub. And don't contaminate yourself again. Got it?" Several of the surgical residents called the medical students "snot." Surgical interns were called "side-boys." All internists and medical residents were call "fleas," implying that they lived on the backs of the surgeons, who were called "top dogs." An alternative term for internists was "feather burner." This implied that medical doctors didn't actually "do" anything, that they only danced around and burned feathers at the bedside.

I was certain I had not touched anything coming into the OR, and positive I had not contaminated myself. I was being hazed, and there was nothing I could do about it. The surgeon in the OR was God, King, Dictator, and Captain of the ship. He had absolute authority. That was the way it was, and I knew it. I slunk into the scrub room and started the re-scrub. Soon little bleeding points appeared on my arms. My skin was now nearly raw. Somehow I got through the repeat scrub, ten full minutes by the clock. Again I backed through the door, taking super extra caution not to touch the door or anything.

I was holding my arms up ready for the circulating nurse to slide the gown onto my hands, when, once again, the surgeon jerked around, looked at me, and said, "I am not going to have some snotty medical student coming in here infecting my patients. You have contaminated yourself again. Scrub another ten full minutes, no fudging. Got it?" He turned to the scrub nurse, "Put the clock on him and let me know when ten minutes is up."

I was fuming. The whole thing was completely unfair. I swung open the door into the scrub room and stood there. I quickly decided that I was not going to scrub again. The case was more than half done. I decided to walk away. I sneaked into the surgeon's dressing room, quickly changed my clothes, and went to the student lab. Hank was pipetting some blood for a white count. I told him what had happened. There was a total of four more weeks on the surgical rotation. I would just hide for the remaining time and do the work on the surgeon's cases if any got assigned to me. Otherwise, I would just not be in contact. I lived in fear of being discovered, but luck was with me, and I made it through undiscovered. I do not think the surgeon ever knew my name. I was able to avoid him for the rest of the month.

The thought of doing surgery for another five years after medical school was unthinkable. Although there are many skills a surgeon needs, there are two minimum qualities for all surgeons—extraordinary physical stamina and the ability to absorb scorn and abuse. I lacked both qualities. After five years of abuse from superiors, it is a miracle surgeons aren't more angry and abusive than some of them are.

In addition to lacking stamina and the ability to absorb verbal abuse, I was just not made to be a surgeon. I did not have the manual dexterity needed to do the work. I did not like to stand for long periods or to hold retractors. I was bored with the very slow progress of most operations. It seemed that opening and closing took hours. But beyond these more physical requirements, I did not think like a surgeon.

Surgeons are action oriented. Their credo is, "Don't just stand there, do something." In contrast, medical physicians might say, "Don't just stand there, do nothing." Surgeons are trained to make decisions on scanty data. Once they decide, they take action. They operate. A surgeon is happiest in the OR. "A chance to cut is a chance to cure" was the antithesis of what I thought was at the heart of medicine.

Surgeons are a special breed, probably identifiable by age five, or at least by the early teens, and most certainly from the first year of medical school. I have taught medical students for more than forty years, and I think I can spot the young surgeons when I first meet them as freshmen. If they played football, they were nearly always a running back, quarterback, or wide receiver—except for the orthopedic surgeons who usually played offensive line.

When my first clinical rotation of the junior year ended, I had already scratched off one career option. Pediatrics, obstetrics, and medicine were still to come.

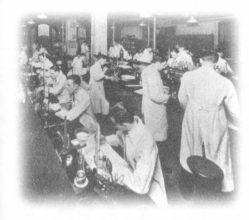

16

SOME LESSONS DO NOT NEED REPEATING

340. Surgery — The object of the course is to instruct the student in those methods of physical diagnosis particularly referable to surgical diseases. The student is instructed in the methods of physical examination of the abdomen, spine, joints, deformities, and other areas of the body.

Catalogue for 1953–1954, page 89
School of Medicine
Vanderbilt University

I WAS ROTATING ON GENERAL SURGERY AS A JUNIOR student, and had been assigned to Rupert Mullins. Mr. Mullins was completely demented and incapable of giving any accurate history. He rambled on about his farm and his daughter, Rheet, with whom he lived. Rheet would show up from time to time to visit. From her, I pieced together her father's full medical history.

Mr. Mullins had been a tobacco farmer with a small patch of acreage in one of the surrounding rim counties. His wife had died about a year before, and he continued to live with his spinster daughter on the same farm. Both were on some sort of welfare, with no other income since Mr. Mullins had been sick. Rheet had to ride the bus to visit her father or catch rides into town with a neighbor. They had no phone, electricity, or running water.

Mr. Mullins had been admitted after falling down the back steps and breaking his hip. His hip had been stabilized, and he had been convalescing in the hospital for more than a month when he was assigned to me. Long hospital stays were common in those days since there were no alternatives—no nursing homes, no home health care, and no rehabilitation units. His daughter had no way to care for him until he became more mobile.

Each night, Mr. Mullins would become more confused, loud, and at times combative. This nocturnal confusion is called the "sundowner syndrome." When the sun goes down, some hospitalized people lose all familiar references in their surroundings and become overtly combative and confused by the shadows and dim light. Every night the staff tied him down at the wrists and ankles. The restraints intensified his confusion, and he would scream out. Every night there was a continual effort to keep him in bed and restrained. The poor lone nurse and one aide, with thirty other patients, had their hands full. The whole scene recalled the Frankenstein movies of my youth, where the mob thinks they have the monster corralled and tied up. In the very next scene and unbeknownst to the town people, the monster begins to untie himself in the basement of the castle.

Late one night, I was sitting at the nursing station writing up my admissions for the day. The ward had been darkened, and the hallway lights were dimmed low. There was light only at the nursing station, where the charge nurse and I sat. We were the only staff present when I heard a commotion down the hall. Mr. Mullins came limping out into the nearly dark hall.

"Rheet, Rheet, for God's sake come git me. They done tied me down. Rheet . . . Rheet . . . come on out the field." His call was loud and plaintive.

Somehow, he had untied the restraints on his arms and legs. He still had the white cloths dangling from his feet and hands. He was stark naked except for the white restraints and the Ace bandages on both legs. He had a long tube attached to his Foley catheter. The tube ran down between his legs and lay out behind him like a string. There was a urine bag still attached to the tubing, being dragged along on the floor several feet behind him. He reminded me of a World War I soldier who had been blown out of the trenches with nothing but his leggings on. This scene was repeated night after night. Nothing the nurses did could keep him in bed.

For some time the intern had been concerned about Mr. Mullins's failure to have a bowel movement. Despite trials with a variety of increasingly strong laxatives, Mr. Mullins had not had a stool in two weeks and had developed a fecal impaction. Fecal impactions were the most dreaded of developments for medical students. First of all, they were completely preventable and were deemed errors in medical management. Second, an impaction would trigger "domino delegation." Upon discovery, the head resident would harangue the junior resident, who would push it off on the intern, who would then "teach" the medical student how to remove the impaction. I was the last domino. There it was, written on the student's yellow sheet, "Remove impaction ASAP and don't let this happen again!" This would be my first experience with a fecal impaction, and I dreaded it.

The next morning I approached Jane Corvil, an instructor from the nursing school, for help. Jane had graduated a year earlier and had dated one of my classmates. She thought it was wonderful that I was going to remove an impaction. Calling it a "teachable moment," she said she wanted her four nursing students to learn about impactions. Whatever she wanted to call it was fine by me. "You know the old saying, 'See one, do one, teach one,'" she said in her unusually cheerful voice. I welcomed her offer to help.

"Miss Corvil," as I called Jane on the ward, had everything set up for me. We were quite formal then, calling each other "Miss" and "Doctor," especially in front of patients and student nurses.

Mr. Mullins was in one of the four-bed rooms down the hall from the large sixteen-bed ward. They kept all the demented patients in the four-bed ward, which kept them sequestered from the other patients. When I walked into the room, the four nursing students had already pulled the curtain and prepared Mr. Mullins for the procedure.

The nursing students stood two on each side of the bed. They had on starched white aprons over light-blue starched dresses, with little white caps pinned to their hair. Little tufts of hair hung down from the backs of their necks. For a moment my mind shifted. I was standing in a garden filled with lilies and hyacinths and rosebuds. The smell of perfume and powder filled the air with the aroma of roses and a hint of jasmine. For the briefest of moments, I was standing in a garden with four beautiful girls at their peak of adolescent beauty.

Jane Corvil stood at the head of the bed, patting Mr. Mullins's head and smoothing his hair, like a mother with her child before an operation.

This was my first time directing nursing assistants, and I felt like a surgeon about to do an important surgical procedure. This was my team, and Miss Corvil was my charge nurse. My team was ready. I felt a sense of command. Despite the context, I mused, this must be how a surgeon feels when he enters a room filled with scrub nurses and assistants. The student nurses stepped back slightly as I entered the curtained-off bed. The perfume intensified.

"Dr. Meador," Miss Corvil said. I could feel my face flush ever so slightly on being called "doctor" by someone my own age. "Dr. Meador, please tell the class what procedure you are going to perform."

Though caught a bit off guard, I was determined to make the most of the opportunity. "Well, I am going to manually enter my finger into the rectum and digitally remove the fecal impaction until I remove all that I can palpate. This procedure should not take long." I had no idea what she wanted me to say, so I put all the big words I could into my effort. "I will need Mr. Mullins in the knee chest position, please."

With some effort, all four student nurses, Jane, and I pulled Mr. Mullins onto his knees. He was nearly limp. It took two student nurses on each side leaning against his body to keep him up on his chest and knees. One student on each side held onto his knees to keep them from slipping back. The other two braced to hold his chest down on the bed. This allowed full access to his rectum. Also, the two nurses closest would be able to have a full view of the "operative site," as I was now calling the area.

As I pulled on the rubber gloves and lubricated the rectal area, I maintained what I hoped was a professional tone, describing for the nurses each step as I did it. Mr. Mullins did not share my professional detachment. On entry into his rectum, he screamed, "For God's sake, Rheet, come he'p me, Rheet!" His screaming got louder and louder.

"Rheet, they killing me, Rheet. Come on out the field. Come on to the house. They got me . . . here . . . now . . . Rheet, Rheet, don't leave me."

I was beginning to sweat. All I could feel was concrete—as hard as any cement I ever felt. I dug and dug with my finger, and, little by little, extracted one small piece after another, letting each one fall into a metal basin between Mr. Mullins's legs. Each one hit the metal bowl like a rock.

Each digging brought more yells. "Stop. Stop. You killing me!"

Suddenly everything changed. At first, I could not figure out what had happened. I felt a sudden hot *something* hit my chest. Then there was an explosion of foul hot liquid. A torrent shot up my sleeve, underneath my shirt, and onto my bare chest. I could feel it running down my chest into my pants. *Oh my God, I've ruptured his aorta,* was my first thought. Then I realized I had hit a pocket of liquid feces. In a seemingly unending torrent, two weeks of failed laxatives worked their way past the broken dam. I tried to stem the flow, but it was no use.

I pulled back, hoping it would stop, but it kept coming like water from a dropped fire hose, spewing out onto the bed and onto the floor. My entire body was drenched with steaming hot liquid feces. I then made the error of all errors: I put the palm of my hand against his rectum hoping to dam up the flow of feces. It did the opposite. My hand created a spewing spray, sending the feces outward and directly onto the student nurses. As the student nurses backed away, Mr. Mullins fell sideways into the pool now filling the bed.

Strangely, in the midst of the screaming and spewing, I was aware of the other three patients in the room shuffling toward the door of the ward. All visitors were gone within seconds. The ward emptied. There we stood. The student nurses were splattered with feces, their starched white and blue uniforms ruined. They still looked like flowers, only now they were long dead and putrid in a vase. I was covered in feces from my shoulders down to my shoes. Jane Corvil, who had stood by the head of the bed, escaped.

The student nurses started to cry. They held their hands out to their sides and shook them in little circles, not knowing what else to do. I wanted to cry, but medical students don't cry. Not ever. I stood there for a moment. The only sounds were the moans of Mr. Mullins and the whimpering of the student nurses. All efforts at professional discourse were abandoned. The students continued to weep as we moved Mr. Mullins into a chair and removed all the sheets and bedclothes. Strangely, even Mr. Mullins had gone silent, too. As I left, I could hear Miss Corvil trying to comfort the students.

I wandered out into the hall still dazed and found a bathroom. I cleaned my face and hands and threw my lab coat into the trash can. My clothes were soaked down my entire front. My shoes squished when I walked. I borrowed a long white coat and started the two-block trudge to the Phi Chi house. I wondered if I would ever be clean again.

I walked down the street and imagined myself packing, calling a cab, getting on the train, and going home. Why should I work eighty to one hundred hours a week to end up like this? I became determined to quit, to leave, to forget the dream. I wanted out. I did not want to spend my life cleaning up feces. If this was medicine, I wanted no part of it.

When I got to the Phi Chi house, I threw all my clothes into the garbage can and walked naked up the stairs to the shower. I scrubbed and re-scrubbed. No matter how long or hard I washed, the fecal odor seemed to remain. I sat on the floor of the shower and let the hot water run over me. I sat there a long time.

There is nothing quite like an explosion of shit to dampen desire and ambition. It was the lowest of low points. After some time, the faces of all those who knew I was studying to be a doctor began to drift across my mind. First my father, then my dead mother, then my brother, my doctor/uncle Sam, and then old Dr. Stabler, my childhood idol. Every teacher or grown-up who knew I was going to be a doctor came into my mind. What would I tell them? How could I tell them that I was quitting because a fecal impaction had exploded in my face? Gradually, the weight of the indignity I had suffered began to lessen, my loss of face before the nursing students faded. This was the only time in four years of medical school that I ever considered quitting.

I dressed and headed back to the hospital. I ran into Hank in the hall. "You won't believe what just happened to me," I said, already thinking about how I would get the most out of the story.

In the fifty years following, I never let another patient get impacted. Some lessons do not need repeating.

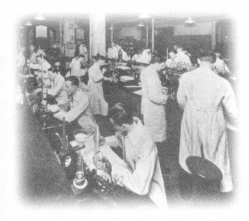

17

A SPECIAL
BREED

1. Pediatric Lectures and Demonstrations. — The prenatal period, the newborn child, mental and physical growth and development, the nutrition of infants and children, and the prevention of the abnormal are discussed. Especial attention is given to the normal child as a basis for the study of the abnormal, or diseases of children. One hour a week during the third trimester of the third year.

2. Ward Work. — One sixth of the third-year class as clinical clerks assigned to the pediatric wards during one half of each trimester. Bedside instruction is given and patients are studied, emphasis being laid on the structure and function of the normal child. Physical diagnosis and variations from the normal and their prevention are considered. Eighteen hours a week during half of one trimester of the third year.

Catalogue for 1953–1954
School of Medicine
Vanderbilt University

IN SURGERY, I LIKED THE CLINICAL SURGICAL PROBLEMS of the patients, but I did not like the abusive style of the surgeons. The opposite was true in pediatrics. I liked the pediatricians, but I did not like the problems involved in caring for the pediatric patients, especially babies.

I could not adjust to the near absence of any history. A child only knows something in a global sense. They are either fine, or they are sick. When they are sick, they have no idea where or what sickness they have. Nearly every disease causes vomiting. With ear infections, they vomit.

With pneumonia, they vomit. Bad tonsillitis, they vomit. You name it, and it causes the child to vomit. Vomiting is a clue for almost nothing.

Ask a child what is bothering him, and he will say, "Just sick," or "Feel bad," or "Nothing, just not good." "Not good" is the state of sickness for most children. Ask a child where he hurts, and he will point at the strangest places. Life is either fine, or it is bad. No shades of gray, no subtle symptoms as in adults. No chance to explore the subtleties of the symptoms or make deductions from them. It is all physical examination combined with the story told by the mother. It is veterinary medicine practiced on humans, and that is not a put-down. To be a pediatrician takes a special person with very special talents.

Children get well incredibly fast. That was one aspect of pediatrics I enjoyed. Down near death one day, up running and playing the next. Pediatrics, especially for infants and toddlers, was as different from adult medicine as it was possible to be. It was not just a specialty of medicine; it was a whole other field. There is an old saying that pediatrics is not internal medicine on little people. It's not even from the same planetary system as internal medicine.

The physical examination of babies and toddlers was nearly impossible, and always difficult for me. It was a fight to get it done. The little patient is holding on to his or her mother, screaming, crying, withdrawing, pulling away, and grabbing at the stethoscope. Ear exams in particular were difficult. By the time I was just beginning to figure out the anatomy of the ear drum, the baby jerked sideways, and I would get lost in the ear canal. Listening to the heart, which was difficult in cooperative adults who could hold their breath, was virtually impossible in an infant who was crying. It was cry, inhale a breath, hear two heartbeats, exhale and scream, inhale, hear two heartbeats, exhale and scream. About all I could tell was that there was a heart present, and even that was a guess.

Dr. Amos Christie was chairman of pediatrics, and he amazed all of us with his ability to examine babies, especially their hearts. In some magical way, he calmed the children and was able to get them to be still. He often let the child sit in the lap of the mother when he did his examination.

The children almost never cried. This was all the more amazing because Dr. Christie was a huge looming figure. He was an All-American tackle on the Washington team that won the Rose Bowl in the 1930s. He looked the part. That was in the days before defensive and offensive teams. All players played the full sixty minutes both ways. Sometimes in his lectures, he would hold a baby in one of his enormous hands and raise the child above his head for all of us to see. He was some huge Greek god come down to earth to teach us about caring for children.

In addition to being a large man, Dr. Christie attracted a faculty large in talent. Four of the six full-time faculty members who taught us went on to be chairmen of pediatrics departments. Floyd Denny was to become chairman at North Carolina; Ralph Petersen at Marquette; Robert Merrill at Arkansas; and Harris (Pete) Riley at Oklahoma. The other two members of the full-time faculty were Randy Batson, who became dean of the School of Medicine at Vanderbilt, and Mildred Stahlman, who went on to literally form the new field of neonatal medicine. More than twenty of Christie's residents would go on to become chairmen of departments of pediatrics. It was quite a department, and Dr. Christie was quite a chairman.

I recall one baby who continued to cry when Dr. Christie was listening to the heart. The child was very sick with bacterial endocarditis, an infection of the heart valve. He went on to describe in detail the location and intensity of the murmurs he heard. He then described how he could feel the vibrations, called "thrills," of the murmur on the chest wall. Each of us in our small group took a turn listening and feeling the chest wall. All I heard was the crying of the child. All I could feel were the vibrations of crying.

Procedures such as drawing blood or starting I.V. fluids were very different from those on adults. Surface veins on the arms or legs are nonexistent in babies, and when found, they are minute. One night I assisted the pediatric intern in starting an I.V. on a small baby. The baby was only a few months old, and the only site for the I.V. was in a scalp vein. I could see the tiny veins running across his bald head. We had to wrap the baby in sheets and then roll him up into a tight bundle to immobilize him. The nurse held the baby on the exam table while the intern tried one small vein after another. The size of the needle was minute, and it took more than an hour to get the needle in a vein that would work. The baby never stopped crying and screaming.

Drawing blood was a difficult process. These days, most of the blood tests can be done on drops of blood from a needle stick in the finger or heel of a baby. No problem. Not so in the 1950s. The tests required larger amounts of blood, necessitating withdrawing blood from larger veins. There were only two sites: the femoral vein in the groin or the external jugular vein in the neck. If those sites failed, it meant going for the deep internal jugular, a scary process. Both were brutal processes to watch. Fortunately for the babies and me, only the interns were allowed to do these procedures. It still amazes me that there were so few complications from such invasive procedures.

One of the biggest differences between pediatrics and adult medicine is the attention paid to the growth and development of children. Children are moving targets. Adults stay about the same from month to month. No one set of norms can be applied to a growing child. The pediatrician uses growth and development for nearly every judgment at every age. Is the child on schedule? At what age did he roll over, sit up, crawl, or walk? What manual manipulations can he perform? Can he stack blocks? Is his mental function and development on schedule? When did he say words or form sentences? The pediatrician is constantly on the alert for any deviation from these stages of early life. Serious chronic diseases usually slow the growth curve. Rare diseases such as hyperthyroidism can accelerate it briefly.

There was one experience alone that may have been the final determining factor driving me away from pediatrics—we called it the Polio Unit. Although the Salk vaccine was under trial, poliomyelitis, then called infantile paralysis, was still common, with frequent summer epidemics. Complete paralysis occurred in the bulbar form of the disease, and death resulted from an inability to breathe if ventilation was not supported mechanically. At the center of the Polio Unit were the rooms for the iron lungs, three to a room. The patients lay inside the devices, enclosed except for their heads. A tight rubber collar was fitted around their neck. Air was pumped out of the iron lung to make the patient's chest expand and thus pull air in. Air was then forced back into the iron lung to make the chest deflate, thus causing the patient to exhale. These large devices were long metal barrels with little locked windows and doors down both sides. Each small window had a rubber cuff to fit around the arm to prevent air from leaking in or out of the opening while the nurses reached in. These provided access to the patient for bathing, changing clothes, and dealing with toilet needs. The rooms reeked of urine and feces despite the constant and diligent attention of the nurses. There is just no way to deal effectively with the toilet needs of children encased in a steel tank.

Iron lungs saved many lives and supported the quadriplegic patients until they regained enough neurological function to breathe unassisted, but there was a tragic side. Many children never came out of the iron lungs. Some lived there for months or even years until they died from a variety of complications. I could not make myself detach emotionally from the pain and agony I saw in the faces of the parents of those children who had given up all chances for a normal life. It was more than I could do.

There was one final thing about pediatrics that turned me away. I could never get used to my patients urinating, defecating, or vomiting on me. Certainly, I had endured the indignity of the fecal impaction episode, but that was one patient and a circumstance I could avoid. Not so in pediatric practice. Nearly every day I was hit with urine, especially from male babies. It was an occupational hazard I could not avoid if I went into pediatrics. I just had to face the facts. I did not have the temperament, skills, patience, or imperturbability required to be a pediatrician. Most of all, I lacked the ability to detach from the emotional pain of seeing a sick and helpless child. Pediatricians are a special breed. They are among the last real doctors remaining. They are the best of all of us, as doctors and as humans.

So I had removed one more career path. Obstetrics was my next rotation.

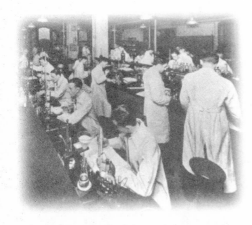

18

Bomber Pilots of Medicine

3. Clinical Obstetrics. — During one half of a trimester a small group of students study the patients on the obstetrical wards and in the outpatient service. They work in the prenatal clinic, practice pelvimetry, and are given exercises with the obstetrical manikin.

During this period students are required to serve as clinical clerks to the obstetrical patients in the hospital and take part in their delivery under the supervision of the staff. All students are required to have assisted in a specified number of deliveries, in the hospital, before graduation.

Approximately eighteen hours a week during a half of trimester of the third year, exclusive of deliveries.

Catalogue for 1953–1954
School of Medicine
Vanderbilt University

ONE OF THE PURPOSES OF THE CLINICAL CLERKSHIPS IN the third year was to allow us to begin to make decisions about our future careers. I had already rejected both pediatrics and surgery. Obstetrics was next.

In obstetrics, more than in any other field, the personality and character of the physicians are intertwined with the character and setting of the patients they see. Obstetricians were the happiest people in the medical school, maybe in all of medicine. I never met one who was a cynic. They, like surgeons, were born and not made.

That kind of enthusiasm and eternal optimism would be impossible to learn.

Other characteristics set obstetricians apart from the pediatrician, surgeons, and other specialists in medicine. They were not deeply concerned with physiology, biochemistry, or the subtleties of the mechanisms of disease. After all, there is nothing subtle about trying to get a seven-pound object through a four-inch opening. Pregnancy is a natural event and can hardly be called a disease. That is, until something goes wrong.

Pregnancy does represent a considerable physiologic upheaval. However, if the body of the woman is sound and a reasonable amount of common sense is applied, the vast majority of women (and husbands, too) come through it with no problems. However, when trouble does come, it is monumental and potentially lethal. There is nothing sicker and more tricky than a woman with a complicated pregnancy and the problem delivery that often accompanies it. Obstetricians are like the bomber pilots of World War II going for a target deep inside Germany. Hours of boring flying, droning toward a distant target. Then fifteen minutes of anti-aircraft flak and chaos, and all hell with machine gun fire while over the target, then hours of droning back to the home field. Obstetrics is 99 percent boredom and 1 percent sheer panic. The rare complications turn the delivery room from a place of friendly chatter and jokes into a place of all-out action in a life or death struggle.

Obstetricians are trained for the 1 percent panic, but none of them really like it. Almost all other fields of medicine warm to the complex and complicated. Nature's rejects and errors are the rest of medicine's major concerns. Not so for obstetrics. Obstetricians prefer the calm routine of a normal delivery. They get their rewards from a warm rapport with the mother, from seeing a healthy new baby brought into the arms of a new mother, and from hearing the *oohs* and *aahs* of the grandparents. Obstetricians are happy people who like to be around happy people. There is no happier place in the world than the room of a new mother on the day after a normal routine delivery. There is no sadder or more depressed place than the meeting of an obstetrician with a family following the birth of a dead or malformed infant. This is human tragedy at its full depth.

There are only a few complications that generate the 1 percent panic—placenta previa (a placenta covering the outlet of the uterus, often associated with bleeding); abruptio placenta (premature separation of the placenta from the wall of the uterus, also associated with bleeding); and a prolapsed cord (umbilical cord preceding the baby). All three are potentially lethal for the baby. Placenta previa and abruptio placenta can also be fatal for the mother. No bomber crew goes into more action than the obstetrical crew when any one of these three complications occurs in the delivery room. All three are equivalent to the heaviest flak and machine-gun fire of air warfare.

As third-year medical students, hungry for the abnormal and severe, we were forced to involve ourselves with the 99 percent of obstetrics that was routine and boring. Unless you loved it and enjoyed working along with a natural process, it quickly drove many of us into another field. Hank was immediately bored, detesting OB as much as I did orthopedic surgery. Every day on the service was a torment for him. He complained every day.

The chairman of obstetrics required us to stay at the bedside of the pregnant woman for the entire period of labor. He said it would allow us to observe the whole process from beginning to end. We were required to feel and record the timing and the length and strength of every uterine contraction. Sometimes we were there by the bedside for twelve to eighteen hours. We became experts at palpating and timing the contracting uterus. Five decades later, I am yet to find any other situation in which to apply that skill.

Finally, with the woman ready to deliver, we moved into the delivery room. I could not get over the extremely good job nature did in lubricating for the event. The slippery tissues in the dog lab and in surgery felt like friction tape compared to every part of the delivery process. Every bit of the apparatus—baby, umbilical cord, and placenta—seemed to be drenched in high-grade machine oil. The amount of liquid that comes with a delivery is huge—several quarts of amniotic fluid, water, and blood. I could not believe it when I first saw a gush cover the delivery room floor. I could not imagine anyone wanting a home delivery. Picture all of that on some kitchen floor or in a bedroom.

After observing a few unbelievable exits of babies from the narrow birth canal, I was convinced that there was not one drop of unnecessary lubrication. My constant fear was that I would either drop the slippery baby or scoot it across the room like a wet melon seed. Obstetricians are born with suction cups for fingers.

In both surgery and pediatrics, nurses obviously play a very important role, but nothing like the nurses in the delivery room. Every medical student who ever hung around a delivery room soon learns that interns, residents, and even obstetricians are just added frills. Nurses are the real force. The head obstetrical and delivery room nurse is a special species. For us, she came in the form of Miss Mabel Atkins. Miss Atkins weighed in at about two hundred and fifty pounds, with a bosom to match. In a scrub suit, which is the only way I ever saw her dressed, she was the benchmark for the yet to come bra-less look.

Somewhere along the line, Miss Atkins had spent ten years in the Army Nurse Corps during and after World War II. Hank and I argued over what she had done in the military. We couldn't decide whether she was in charge of shooting deserters or whether she led the troops ashore at Anzio. She could out-cuss and out-yell even the filthiest-mouthed resident. Except for her time in the Army, she had spent all of her career in a delivery room. No one could smoke a cigarette or hold a coffee mug with more authority than Miss Atkins. She was master sarge and nose gunner combined.

Always feigning boredom and nonchalance, she paid us almost no attention. Medical students were seen by her for just what we were— young, green students who knew nothing and who could only get in her way. I gave her plenty of room and never talked to her unless she spoke to me first. Before our rotation was over, we came to be friends of a sort. She even liked Hank. She said at least we kept our mouths shut. That must have been her highest compliment. She was an encyclopedia of obstetrics, but not one that would be literature referenced. She had seen it all. I learned most of the obstetrics I know from her. The residency program would have collapsed without her.

Miss Atkins was a chain smoker. One time she knocked off half a cigarette in one drag. I was afraid the thing would burst into flames before she quit pulling. Labor, to Miss Atkins, was an event that transpired between cigarette drags. Laying the lit butt down on her desk, she ran in and out of the labor rooms checking on each patient. Her desk top was charred with little black marks from years of forgotten burning butts.

Miss Atkins would sit in the small office-lounge just outside the delivery rooms. The six labor rooms ran down the hall beside the office-lounge. It was there that Miss Atkins guzzled her constant coffee, took drags on her cigarettes, and listened for the sounds coming from the labor rooms. Most of the patients we saw were indigent, poorly educated, and deeply religious—at least during labor. Miss Atkins used the religious fervor of the patients to her advantage for following the stages of labor.

Labor progresses by steady, relentless dilatation of the uterine cervix. As the baby's head pushes down into the pelvis, the cervix opens a bit more with each contraction. As labor intensifies, the contractions become more and more forceful and painful. Starting at one centimeter, the cervix dilates to a full ten centimeters (about four inches) in diameter at the time of delivery. In those days, most obstetricians, residents, medical students, and other nurses followed the stages of labor by examining the cervix via repeated rectal examinations (the cervix can be felt through the rectal wall). Miss Atkins had a different method.

Miss Atkins followed the calls and cries of the women. The uneducated and fundamentally religious background of the patients worked to Miss Atkins's advantage. This was not a racial or ethnic thing. We saw patients from both races. It was more deeply rural, religious, and Southern than racial. When the pitch, hue, and content of the cries got just right, she wheeled the woman into the delivery room, got everything ready, and then called the resident and obstetricians. She was never wrong. Whenever Miss Atkins called, you could bet that labor was full blown and the cervix fully dilated. The residents and obstetricians loved her.

I learned bits and pieces of her methods, although I missed many of the subtleties.

"Oh, Lawd. Lawdee," was a cervix of no more than one or two centimeters. Early labor at best. The patient would repeat the phrase or some equivalent with each contraction in a bored or sleepy voice. Sighs or deep breathing followed, and the patient often fell back asleep. Each patient had a canister of Trilene gas with a mask strapped to her wrist. They could breathe this if the pain got too bad. The mask fell away from the face, making it safe to use.

"Lawdee, Lawdee, Lawdee," said in a crescendo, usually meant four or five centimeters of dilatation and the beginning of steady labor. The pitch was higher and definitely not bored or sleepy.

"Lawdee, Lawdee, Sweet Jeeee-sus," came with seven or eight centimeters, loud but not the full volume of a fully dilated cervix or imminent delivery.

"Lawdee Jeeee-sus. He'p me. He'p me, sweet Jeee-sus. Sweet Jeesus, save me." The cry was full volume and shrill. There was an undeniable urgency about it—full of demand for help—and soon.

I facetiously wondered how private delivery rooms ever staged labor. I suspect Miss Atkins would not have been as finely tuned in an OB service in some full pay private hospital.

Obstetrics came and finally passed. It was not for me. Each new rotation picked off a few classmates who thought they had found their life's work. I believe I could have picked out the future jovial obstetricians before medical school. Several of our happiest chose OB. The young surgeons were already clearly identifiable. By now Hank was a hopeless case and in love with surgery. A few of the class had decided on pediatrics. A very few, three to be exact, chose psychiatry. The rest of us were still looking. The clerkship in medicine was next.

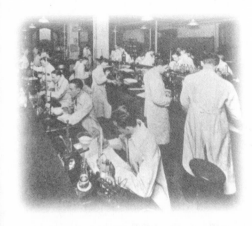

19

MEDICINE
AT LAST

3. Ward Work. — One-third of the third year class is assigned to the medical wards during each quarter and one-half during a quarter of the summer term. Here they serve as clinical clerks. In this assignment they become part of the team of resident, assistant resident, intern, attending physician, and chief of the service responsible for the diagnostic study and treatment of patients. Bedside instruction is given daily by members of the staff who are also members of the faculty. Approximately 20 hours a week during one quarter.

Catalogue for 1953–1954
School of Medicine
Vanderbilt University

THE LAST CLINICAL ROTATION OF THE THIRD YEAR FINALLY came. Internal medicine at last. I had been tormented and humiliated by the surgeons. I had been bewildered by the near absence of patient histories in pediatrics. I had endured the boredom of obstetrics. Internal medicine was like coming home after a long, trying journey.

Internal medicine was the largest of puzzles. Nearly every patient represented a fascinating detective story. At the end of an evening's work, I would read about the diseases I had seen that day. The next morning I could hardly wait to look for the subtle points I had read about the night before.

Internal medicine is as broad in scope as human illness itself. It is not limited to technique as in surgery, narrowed to certain reproductive organs as in obstetrics, or restricted by age range group as in pediatrics. Internal medicine excludes no organ. It calls on the widest possible look at a patient. One must see the forest, the trees, and all that lies between and beyond them. As internists, we would learn to consider the patient's occupation and workplace, the substances he ingested, the air he breathed, and even substances he rubbed on or rubbed against. We would need to develop, whether through inquiry or intuition, the ability to detect when the patient's very family or friends might be contributing to the illness. Medicine called on physiology, biochemistry, pathology, and all of the other subjects we had learned. It was an integration of all fields on a grand scale.

I, like many internists I would come to know, was a fan of Sherlock Holmes. As teenagers, a friend and I would sit on the curb downtown and try to guess the occupations of the passersby from their dress or gait or from their shoes. We bantered in our make-believe of Watson and Holmes.

In medical school, I learned to look for small clues. Internal medicine was the home of faint signs that led to larger diagnoses. I looked at fingers and hands for calluses or clubbing, or for the nicotine stains of the smokers, or the chewed nails of the anxious. I looked at the soles of shoes for uneven worn spots, often clues to limps or neurological problems. I looked at the belts for changing notches that might give away increases or decreases in abdominal girth or weight. The color of stains on underclothing could often tell of unknown blood in the urine or stool or even the unmistakable yellow stains of jaundice. I became a student of breath odors—the stench of old whiskey, the overly perfumed secret alcoholic woman, the fruity smell of acetone, the fetor of liver failure, the ammonia of renal failure, or the putrid odor of a lung abscess. I never got as good as Holmes, but he was my model.

This attention to small details was not just a medical student exercise. We had to make diagnoses from the history and physical examination. Screening tests were unheard of. The tests we used were not yet as specific or sensitive as those we now have. There were a few tests for liver function. Except for the EKG, a measure of circulation time, and a crude measure of venous pressure, there were no precise tests for cardiac function. The vital capacity for lung function was all we had. Blood gases were still available only in the research laboratory. The brain was examined by the neurological examination or a plain skull X-ray, which sometimes showed a calcified pineal gland if the patient was lucky. Lateral shifts of the calcified pineal indicated mass lesions. The electroencephalogram (EEG) was just being understood.

Since we lacked sensitive diagnostic tools, we operated in a world of far advanced diseases. Early disease, especially early chronic disease, was unusual to see and difficult to diagnose. Kampmeier had told us that anyone can find far advanced disease; it took a real doctor to find early disease.

Learning internal medicine required seeing and hearing as many patients and as much disease as possible so we could draw on this catalog of experience when we needed it later. I learned that we see only what we look for. The more I could see in medical school, the more I would know to look for in my future patients. We made every effort to see each other's patients—to listen to the different murmurs, to feel enlarged spleens, to listen to the rales and other signs of pneumonia, to see jaundice and know that artificial lighting could hide it, to learn to detect the faint blueness of cyanosis, and to feel an encyclopedia of abdominal masses.

Hank hated medicine as much as I disliked surgery. He disliked the inaction, the waiting, and the long drawn-out period of observing to see what might surface with time. Time to a surgeon is the next five minutes. Time to an internist can be the greatest diagnostician. He was frustrated in making a diagnosis when nothing could be done about it. He could not abide chronic disease, with its slow relentless course and only the small adjustments medicine could make. These frustrations were common to all surgeons—past, present, and future. For Hank, the embodiment of his frustration with medicine came alive in Dr. Elliot Newman.

Elliot Newman was the first of the new wave of clinical scientists who began to re-populate Vanderbilt's School of Medicine faculty in the 1950s. Vanderbilt had fallen from its pre–World War II scientific zenith. The war and recruitment by other medical schools had depleted the faculty of many of its luminaries. Among those who had left were Sidney Burwell, who had gone to be dean of the Harvard Medical School, and Alfred Blalock, to be chairman of surgery at Johns Hopkins. Tinsley Harrison, whose textbook was one of two medical bibles of the day, would found and chair three departments of medicine after he left Vanderbilt: Bowman Gray, Southwestern, and Alabama. Dr. Newman was to lead the rebuilding of clinical sciences at Vanderbilt. Like many who followed and preceded him, he also came from Johns Hopkins.

When he arrived at Vanderbilt in 1952, he was appointed to the newly endowed Werthan Chair of Experimental Medicine, and he initiated a program in clinical investigation. This investigative program expanded and multiplied, eventually leading to the establishment of the National Institute of Health (N.I.H.)–supported Clinical Research Center (CRC) by the late 1950s. Dr. Newman was director of the CRC for many years, building the program to national prominence within a short time.

My most direct contact with Dr. Newman occurred several years after I graduated. I had returned to residency training from the Army medical corps in 1959, and my first rotation was to be on the cardiology service under Dr. Newman. In the few years since my graduation from medical school, Dr. Newman had set up the cardiac catheterization laboratory, established a full-blown pulmonary function lab, expanded the Clinical Research Center, and had begun to create the specialty of cardiology in the department of medicine. Where there had been only one research fellow in the early 1950s, there were now research fellows in several departments. Clinical investigation was a bustling enterprise in many departments of the School of Medicine by the early 1960s.

During my rotation as a resident, Dr. Newman had me abstract all of the charts of patients with atrial septal defects, see the patients when they came to the clinic, and formulate the details of the clinical syndromes associated with these congenital cardiac defects. By the end of the rotation, I had become an expert of sorts on atrial septal defects. It was the first time I ever went to the depths of understanding to such an extent in any subject. The experience gave me a great appreciation for in-depth knowledge and what it takes to internalize that level of knowing.

Hank and I first saw Dr. Newman in our third year. Toward the end of the third year, Dr. Newman was to give a lecture on congestive heart failure. The class ahead of us had warned us that he could be vague, that he was given to long digressions. Some said he appeared lost in thought. These negative opinions of the seniors preceded our first encounter with him and biased many of my classmates.

Dr. Newman ambled into the room. He started the session by having the medical resident present the history and physical findings of a sixty-year-old man who had severe congestive heart failure. Our entire class was present, as was required for these special lectures in medicine, which ran weekly during all of the third year. In those days the patient, accompanied by a student nurse, was always present for any presentation. The man was short of breath even while sitting in his wheelchair. He could only say a few words between breaths. He had massive edema of his legs and a large liver. The veins in his neck were dilated and looked like ropes under his skin. After thanking the patient for coming to the class and having the resident wheel the man into the hallway, Dr. Newman went to the blackboard and wrote, "What is heart failure?"

He opened the lecture with, "Can anyone tell me what congestive heart failure is?" With that opening he stood silently and motionless for several minutes. Hank started shifting in his seat. Hank, becoming increasingly surgical every week, did not like wasted time. He detested most things about internal medicine, especially what he labeled "wool gathering." I could tell it was going to be a long hour for Hank.

"What is congestive heart failure? Anyone care to tell me?" Dr. Newman asked again, his face expressionless. He looked around the room. No one said a word. We had long learned as a class *never* to volunteer. Volunteering usually ended badly for the student. Dr. Newman waited for what seemed an eternity. Then he waited some more. Hank began to squirm.

Completely out of character, Hank blurted out, "It's when the heart can't pump enough blood." He mumbled under his breath (as an aside to me), "Any fool knows that."

"Well, how would we know that?" Dr. Newman asked back, moving around the podium toward the front row.

Hank was now on the spot. "You would hear rales in the lungs; the neck veins would be full, the liver would be enlarged—be palpable; there would be edema of the legs. Things like that." Hank went on to give a full and accurate clinical description of a patient with congestive heart failure.

"I can find all of those things in a combination of diseases— thoracic inflow obstruction, cirrhosis, pneumonia, malnutrition. What is specifically going on in congestive heart failure? You said something earlier about not pumping enough blood? I still don't follow you on that point." Dr. Newman did not change his expression.

"Well, when the heart does not pump enough blood, you get those findings," Hank answered.

Hank was now fully engaged and becoming slightly irritated. Several other classmates began to mumble and move in their chairs.

Another classmate said, "Well, if the heart is failing, it will have a low cardiac output. It can't pump right."

Dr. Newman then went on to tell us that some patients with congestive heart failure actually had higher than normal cardiac outputs. What did we think of that? "So, if the cardiac output can be high in patients with congestive heart failure, what is congestive heart failure if it's not limited to patients with low cardiac output?"

"Maybe the cardiac output is not high enough," another classmate volunteered.

"Then how high should it be? Say, if the cardiac output is, for example, 7.0 liters per minute? Normal being around 3.5." Again, Dr. Newman stood quietly, like he had nothing else to do. He was in no hurry.

The class was now visibly upset. Here we were supposed to get our usual dose of a well-ordered lecture on a subject. And what were we getting but one question after another, all seeming to lead nowhere. Usually the lecturers told us everything to be known on a subject. All the would-be surgeons were rapidly becoming agitated. Hank was turning red in the face.

"Look," Hank said in a very loud voice, "the heart is pumping blood, but not all that it should. The blood backs up; fluid eases out into the lungs, liver, and the body. And that's congestive heart failure."

Dr. Newman listened attentively, then stood silently, obviously deep in thought. His silence only fanned the class irritation.

"You tell us what it is." This came from the back of the room.

"Yeah, you tell us what heart failure is." There were shouts from several classmates.

Dr. Newman smiled faintly. "Well, let's go back to 'but not all the blood it should.' What do you mean by that? It is pumping, say, 7.0 liters per minute and should be pumping 7.1. Is that what you mean?"

"Yeah, yeah." More classmates now joined Hank.

"That's what we mean. Some number higher than 7.0."

"The blood backs up," another called out.

Dr. Newman went to the blackboard and wrote 7.1 minus 7.0 and got 0.1 liter difference. "So, zero-point-one liter of blood per minute is not getting pumped? Right?" The class almost as a whole yelled back, "Yes, that's it."

Newman pulled out a large circular slide rule, which he carried in his white coat. He moved the plastic arms in one direction, then back and then back again. Looking at the slide rule, he began to write more numbers on the board.

"In one minute, there will be point-one liters backed up. My slide rule tells me that in one hour 60 times 0.1 liters equals 6.0 liters. There would be 6.0 liters not pumped in one hour. My slide rule tells me that 6 times 24 equals 144 liters. Therefore, in 24 hours there would be 144 liters not pumped. At some point looks like the patient would explode." Dr. Newman smiled broadly and chuckled to himself, entirely self-satisfied with his little joke.

After some suggestions back and forth, Dr. Newman proved that the heart, even in failure, must pump all the blood presented to it; so congestive heart failure was not as simple as many in the class suggested.

"So, what is congestive heart failure?" he asked once more. We were nowhere in our efforts to define it.

"It's when the venous pressure is high," someone suggested.

"I can list many conditions without heart failure where the venous pressure is high. Any obstruction to the blood inflow into the heart or chest can cause an elevated venous pressure. Constrictive pericarditis is associated with a high venous pressure. So high venous pressure does not define heart failure."

"So, what is congestive heart failure?" Newman again and again returned to his original question. We could describe in detail the clinical findings of heart failure, but we could not define it physiologically. Over the next forty-five minutes, many suggestions were made. "It's when there is a gallop rhythm." "It's when the heart is enlarged." "It's when a patient gets short of breath walking." "It's a state of salt and water retention." Most suggestions were symptoms or physical findings or general derangements in physiology, but not specific for heart failure. Dr. Newman rejected all as not defining the mechanisms involved in a failing heart.

Late in the hour many in the class were beginning to speak in very loud voices, bordering on yelling, "Tell us," or, "Well, what is it?" or "We don't know, you tell us." Hank was disgusted, frustrated, and mumbling to himself.

Dr. Newman stood benignly smiling and nodding, saying nothing. The clock was only a few minutes from the close of the hour.

Dr. Newman folded his notes and started for the door. He spoke back over his shoulder. "I don't know what congestive heart failure is. I only know what it is not." With that, he left the room. The class erupted.

I had never seen my classmates so upset. Privately, I thought the session was a masterpiece of Socratic teaching. Just about every classmate spent the next weeks reading extensively about heart failure. Nothing had ever driven us to read and discuss any subject as much as Dr. Newman did. We learned that there were two dominant theories about congestive heart failure: the forward failure theory and the backward failure theory. We also learned that Tinsley Harrison, now chairman of medicine at Alabama, had done the fundamental clinical and experimental work on congestive heart failure. He had published his now classic "Failure of the Circulation" in 1935, while a member of the faculty of Vanderbilt School of Medicine. Harrison favored the backward theory. By the 1950s, no one had yet reconciled the two theories.

In the fifty years since, that hour with Dr. Newman is still vivid in my memory. It directed my thinking and reading about subjects beyond heart failure even to this day. I consider the session one of the finest teaching hours I have experienced.

Although we could describe in great detail the clinical findings of congestive heart failure, we could not define the altered physiology. Dr. Newman was asking us to define the mechanism that goes into play when the heart fails. As I began to look at other clinical syndromes, it was clear that we knew very little about underlying mechanisms. Dr. Newman taught us to see that we could know at several levels of understanding, but still not know ultimate causation.

Medicine was the promise of the future. We were still very much in the early scientific phase of understanding the human body and its diseases. That was the attraction for me. To be a part of the unfolding of that science was what captured my attention. In a few years we would have the cardiac catheter, blood gases, and varied pulmonary function tests. We would be able to measure sodium and potassium in blood, which we could not do in those years. We would soon have sensitive liver functions tests. And in the more distant future, the whole puzzle of human genetics and DNA would explode onto the scene. Endocrinology and immunology were still in primitive but very exciting phases. Hormones were just beginning to be measured. Cortisone as a drug had come out the year before, and prednisone was to come out the next year. A few antibiotics were available, and more were coming every year.

But none of these promises caught Hank's attention. He was a man of action. Medicine, for people of action, could be vague, dull, and too slow to take action. Knowing the "natural course of a disease," by-words for internists, was anathema to Hank. Surgeons don't permit natural courses if there is anything that can be incised or removed. Internists work with nature whenever possible. To surgeons nature is the enemy; death is their defeat.

The deep philosophic differences between surgeons and internists go back into antiquity. The field of medicine dates to the early Greek temples, and from there to Padua, where the earliest sciences arose. Medicine has its roots in the spiritual and the sacred. This dichotomy carries over to this day. Surgeons call internists "feather burners" to evoke these ancient religious origins.

Surgeons come out of wars. They were there to repair traumas, to amputate mutilated limbs, to drain abscesses, to close wounds, splint fractures, and stop bleeding. There is a necessary urgency in surgery that is not present in much of medicine.

Surgeons will say the internists waited too long to call them. That is sometimes true. Internists will say the surgeons acted too quickly. That, too, is sometimes true. This conflict, while much less present today, will always be present to some degree. The internist prefers to wait. Nature heals. The surgeon prefers to act. A chance to cut is a chance to cure. We need each other, however hard that is to admit.

The third year came to an end. We would begin to look for internships.

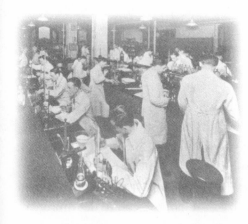

20

STORY
OF A
BLOWN PUPIL

1. Neurological Surgery. — A clinical presentation of neurological problems with emphasis on diagnosis and management.

Catalogue for 1953–1954, page 90
School of Medicine
Vanderbilt University

A STUDENT WHO WAS IN THE CLASS A YEAR AHEAD OF US had developed a bad reputation. I will call him Mort. One of Mort's favorite tricks was to scout the emergency room mid-afternoon. He would find a patient who was about to be admitted. Then he would race to the student assignment sheet and write the patient's name by his name. In this way, he could jump ahead of his classmates and get an early admission, thus finishing his day's work and having the evening off. It infuriated his classmates and anyone who heard about it. His classmates caught him doing it and tried to ostracize him, with no success. Mort was one of those thick-skinned people who are not affected by the opinions of others and who don't care what anyone thinks. Nearly all the medical students hoped Mort would get caught by the faculty in one of his ploys. It finally happened on a neurosurgical patient.

All of the surgical specialties were included in the senior surgical clerkship, where Mort was rotating. This included neurosurgery. We had been taught to stay in the background on neurosurgical patients because of the fast pace whenever one of them turned sour. This was particularly true for patients with head injuries, all of whom were admitted to neurosurgery.

In the 1950s, there were no cerebral arteriograms, certainly no CT scans, or MRIs, or other high-tech noninvasive studies that can nowadays quickly determine the presence, location, and amount of bleeding inside the skull. These devices now provide data that assist the neurosurgeon in deciding who needs to have the skull opened for drainage. Those technical advances would be years in coming. At the time, only careful clinical follow-up by repeated neurological examinations could determine if there was intracranial bleeding that needed surgical evacuation. The clinical evaluations also had to answer the question about the site of the bleeding in the brain. The real clinical trick was to know when to operate and when not to. For some cases of intracranial bleeding, the surgeons watched and waited; for others they operated immediately. Those decisions took years of clinical experience and training. It was why neurosurgical training took seven years beyond medical school. I had great respect for neurosurgeons as clinicians, and still do.

One of the cardinal signs of increasing intracranial pressure is the dilatation of the pupil of one eye. The other pupil remains normal in size. This occurs because of pressure and torsion on the nerve that controls pupil constriction. The dilatation of a single pupil is called a "blown pupil." The appearance of a blown pupil can denote a neurosurgical emergency, especially when the pupil had previously been observed to be normal in size. It is one sign that can lead to immediate drilling into the skull (called "burr holes") to allow blood to escape and to decrease the intracranial pressure. What would be enough bleeding to make a large bruise on an arm can be fatal if it occurs inside the nonexpandable, bony skull.

Mort's patient was a young man admitted following a fall from a horse. Horses and motorcycles generated much of traumatic neurosurgery; they still do, even with the laws requiring helmets. Since the man was an emergency admission, all Mort had to do was to write a summary of the intern's notes.

The man was unconscious, but with no focal neurological signs at the time of admission. His pupils were equal in size and reactive to light. The residents and nursing staff were following him carefully every few minutes. Intensive care units did not exist, so he was in one of the four-bed units where the sicker patients were aggregated. Vital signs were taken every few minutes. In some cases an EKG rhythm strip was also run periodically (continuous monitors were still in the future). A nurse stood by the bedside doing almost constant neuro-checks, as they were called. The neurosurgical house staff and medical students were supposed to hover and watch. It was an intense clinical activity. These patients taught us the details of neurological examina-tions, which, on top of our intensive course in neuroanatomy, prepared us in the basics of assessing neurological problems.

Hank and I were in the cafeteria having a Coke, when Mort ambled up to the table. We wondered why he was in the cafeteria with such a sick new admission. The grapevine was quite active, and we knew immediately about nearly every new admission, including Mort's head trauma case. We tried to ignore Mort until he persisted in inter-rupting us. He told us about his new admission, the young man who fell off of the horse.

He was presenting the findings to us, spewing out all sorts of eponyms for the neurological signs and showing off his knowledge of neuroanatomy. Mort made some wild speculation about some injury to the caudate nucleus or maybe some bleeding into the hippocampus. Hank kept mumbling "bullshit" to each of Mort's theories. Mort then told us about the eye exam. For some reason still unknown and incom-prehensible to anyone, Mort made the unpardonable mistake of dilating one pupil with atropine. When he told us what he had done, Hank and I, in one movement, jumped up from the table and started running toward 3300.

When we got there, we saw a trail of sheets, pillows, and other scat-tered bedclothes coming out of the four-bed unit into the hallway. The young man's bed was empty. We called to the nurse to find out where they had taken him.

The nurse called from the nursing station. "Blown pupil . . . gone to the OR . . . for burr holes."

We wheeled around to find Mort behind us. "You stupid ass," Hank yelled. "Get up to the OR and stop them."

We followed Mort, close behind, half running, hearts pounding, in complete fear of meeting the neurosurgeon, yet wanting to be sure Mort relayed the information so the surgeon would not do unnecessary burr holes. As soon as we saw Mort go into the OR, we ducked out of sight, not wanting any association with Mort or his horrible error.

Joe Capps, who was the chief neurosurgical resident, loved to tell this story. He especially liked to tell it over and over whenever Mort was around. In fact, if Mort ever walked up when Joe was around, Joe would stop what he was saying and immediately tell the story again. Joe said Dr. Bill Meacham, the chief of neurosurgery, on hearing about the one-eyed atropine, collared Mort and pinned him up against the wall. Joe said if they had not pulled Meacham off, he would have punched Mort out. Meacham screamed in Mort's face and cursed him. When he left the OR, Dr. Meacham headed straight to the dean's office to get Mort kicked out of medical school.

We had been told over and over in Hartman's and Kampmeier's courses *never* to dilate neuro patients' eyes for any reason. The size and equality of the pupil was one of the key signs for following the clinical course of all neuro patients. I don't think they ever said not to dilate one eye, but who would have ever thought anyone was stupid enough to do that? Some things don't need to be said.

The young man barely escaped an unneeded burr hole, slowly recovered consciousness, and was discharged in good condition with no residual neurological damage. An unnecessarily shaved head was the only damage done.

For reasons we never heard, Mort was not kicked out of medical school. He must have fast-talked the dean somehow. We never saw any change in Mort's behavior or anything resembling contrition.

If someone is going to be arrogant, they had better be real smart, better yet, brilliant. Only true geniuses can afford to be arrogant, and even then it is an insufferable trait. Mort was smart but far from brilliant. Arrogant people who are not geniuses will inevitably make a glaring mistake. It will not be a simple mistake. It will be huge. Sometimes I wonder if God doesn't look around for arrogant people and punish them by causing them to make stupid errors. Mort's mistake was truly stupid and colossal, yet somehow he escaped punishment.

Of all the causes of malpractice lawsuits I have seen in the years that followed, arrogance in a physician leads the list. The arrogant physician does not listen to other physicians, nor does he listen even to friends or spouse. Seemingly immune to all feedback except one source, the arrogant physician has made the deadly mistake of believing only the high praise of his patients. Nearly all patients pour out praise, and it is a treacherous road to accept it at face value. Undiluted acceptance of patient praise is a constant occupational hazard, and it feeds arrogant physicians. The arrogant physician, who cuts himself off from the honest direct feedback of colleagues and friends, is headed for disaster.

Arrogance follows closely on the heels of the "foot of pride," as the Bible puts it. Eventually, the arrogant physician will exceed his limits of justified professional pride and be kicked into reality. Maybe the dean believed that Mort had learned some important lesson from his mistake. None of us believed he had learned a single thing.

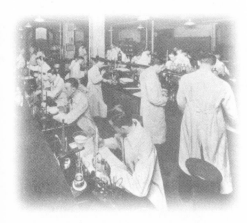

21

Sounds
of Night

*During the third and fourth year, the students continue as clinical clerks and are
assigned in small groups to the various services in the Hospital where they become
junior members of the teams studying problems and progress of patients.*

Catalogue for 1954–1955, page 67
School of Medicine
Vanderbilt University

THE HOSPITAL CHANGED CHARACTER AT NIGHT. ALL OF THE
visitors left, except those with a dying family member. The nursing staff
thinned down to a minimum of one staff nurse and one or two nursing
aides for thirty-two patients. Once the patients were all bedded down,
the nurses gathered at the nursing station to do their charting. There
was a long workbench where we medical students did our write ups, kept
our charts, and plotted the results of our lab work from the day. I especially liked the hospital after midnight. There was a cozy feeling late at
night, particularly if the ward was calm, no one was in critical condition,
and there was no new admission. All the lab work had been done, all the
charting finished, all the notes done for the next day, and all my lab work
slips ready for the next morning. Sitting and half-listening to the women
talk quietly back and forth was somehow reassuring and calming. It
reminded me of nights with my grandmother and great aunt when they
lived in the country, the two old women knitting and talking and rocking
by the light of kerosene lamps as I played on the floor.

Sometimes I wandered out of the ward onto the outdoor walkway that connected 3200 and 3300. The walkway had a tiled floor and a partially covered roof, like an open arbor in a garden or the top deck of a great ship. Cool fall nights were best. If the football stadium lights were not on, the stars came out brilliantly and filled the sky. After the hot stale air of the wards, the cool night air was invigorating. Sweat— a constant in the overheated wards no matter the season—was banished by the coolness. On Saturday nights in the fall, I could see the distant lights of the football stadium and hear the crowd roar wax and wane, depending on how the team was doing. When the game was over and the crowd was heading back to the fraternity houses, I would lean over the stone wall and eavesdrop on the undergraduate students passing by on the sidewalk below. Sometimes I could hear them distinctly talking of the dance to follow the game or pick up some comments about the opposing team, but mostly it was a mumble so low I couldn't catch all the words. I could almost feel the fine hair and smell the paralyzing perfume of some wonderful and beautiful co-ed as she laughed in passing.

Those nights made me realize how far apart we had moved from the other world in such a short time. The other world would only show us the tragic fragments of their sick and injured. Our view would forever be skewed toward the abnormal. The remainder of the other world remained invisible and inaccessible to us. We were separated by the work we did and the things we saw and heard. We would be treated as separated people. Never again would I walk casually to a football game with nothing on my mind except my date and the upcoming game. I sometimes felt a yearning, but those feelings were quickly suppressed, as the urgency of the next I.V. to start or the stat white count to be done or the new admission on the way up from the ER demanded my presence. I liked to sneak out onto those walkways, but even those breaks came infrequently. By the time of internship, they would go away forever.

Around 1:00 A.M., the hospital lights were turned off except in the hallways of the wards. The rest of the hallways were unlighted. The outside appearance of the hospital, as I approached it when called back in the middle of the night, was like a huge ocean liner with rows of lights interspersed with blackness. There were passengers and crew and even a captain. Inside its confines countless smaller voyages were underway, or ending. We were constantly at sea on a ship that never pulled into a port, never docked. Like small boats, ambulances would pull alongside and discharge the bodies damaged by the harshness of life or the misfortunes of disease. They were like rescue boats pulling the sick and wounded out of the ocean. Some of the rescued would eventually make it back to shore, but others would be lost at sea.

One night I was sitting at the bench at the nursing station, finishing the recording of my lab work for the day. As I listened to the sounds of the ward, I began to distinguish one patient from another. There were no women in this ward. They were all on the ward one floor down.

The fat man with congestive heart failure in the far-off left corner of the ward slept sitting up to permit him to breathe. Even then, he snored in long sonorous inspirations occasionally punctuated with abrupt snorts and jerks as he fought to break through his tongue, which periodically obstructed his airway.

The man in one of the front four beds, the one closest to the nursing station, had severe emphysema. His cough was feeble and protracted as he wheezed out only a small amount of air with each cough. He sputtered like a distant motor that wouldn't quite crank. Over and over again, he hawked weakly until he cleared enough mucous to catch a slightly better breath and a few more minutes of sleep.

In the second bed on the right, the World War II veteran with bronchitis had a vigorous cough. It was wet and full of phlegm and mucus and ended in a sputter and hawk. And then quiet.

The faint hiss of oxygen going into the plastic tent of the old man with heart failure merged with the background sounds of bubbling water on the oxygen tank There was a Maws inhaler kettle with the whistle of boiling menthol water close by the nursing station. Off in the distance of the ward, I could hear someone say something to the man in the next bed, then an even fainter and less distinct response, followed by silence. All I could tell was that it was a lone human voice somewhere out on the darkened ward.

I could soon follow each patient by his sound or the absence of a sound. One night the nurse told me that was how she tracked the ward. She had a sense about her when something was not right. She would grab her flashlight and move onto the ward, quickly finding the patient in need through some sixth sense in addition to her keen sense of hearing.

I learned to distinguish the different coughs at night sitting there listening to the sounds of the ward . . . the wet crackling of congestive heart failure, the sputtering protracted ones of chronic bronchitis and emphysema, the faint rattling cough of terminal lung cancer, the raucous honking of cavitary tuberculosis, and the loud and effective coughs of otherwise healthy men with acute pneumonia or influenza.

Nights were full of horrors for some patients, especially those with dementia. Like Rupert Mullins with the impaction, they were able to function in the day, but as soon as the sun went down, they became confused and even combative. Shadows became some attacking beast or worse. The flicker of the nurse's flashlight could trigger a frantic scream. No longer able to see faces or hear familiar voices, they became frightened and lost. Their occasional cries and whimpers blended with the intermittent coughs and other sounds of the night.

In the deep dead of the night, say after 3:00 A.M., the hospital became very quiet, a motionless ship no longer buffeted by waves. The hospital had a lone telephone operator who ran the overhead paging system. After midnight, she turned the volume down low so any paging had to be listened for. Sometimes I could hear her faint snoring over the speaker. She must have slept from time to time. How else could she pass the time with nothing going on for hours at a time in the middle of the night?

It was at the bottom of the night that Mazie made her rounds. Mazie was a very old black woman who had been a part of the hospital since it opened in 1925. Every evening after midnight, Mazie made a large urn of coffee, which she pushed on a cart from one ward to another to give the nurses a much needed boost in the middle of the night.

Coffee would wake me quickly, but I could not go to sleep afterwards. I was very sensitive to caffeine. One night I was in the kitchen on the ward looking around for something to eat. All of the food had been eaten, but I found a jar of unsweetened grapefruit juice. I drank down a glass of the stout stuff. In seconds, I was wide awake from the jolt. From then on, I used unsweetened grapefruit juice to keep me awake on long nights.

Late one night, well after midnight, Mazie had just passed through the ward where I was writing up a patient's history. The very faint voice of the operator came over the speaker system. At first it was like a hoarse whisper, and I could not make it out. Then nothing. Then a faint whisper coming from the operator.

"Mazie. Mazie. Where are you, Mazie?" the operator whispered over the speaker.

Then several minutes later, this time a little louder, "Mazie, where are you? Mazie. Mazie?"

Several more minutes passed, and then in a loud mid-day voice with the volume turned up, the operator demanded, "MAZIE, I NEED COFFEE. NOW!"

I can still hear the desperation in the operator's voice and understand it.

When a very sick patient was admitted late, the night changed quickly, and time vanished. The pink light of dawn was there before I knew it. At first blinded by the bright light of day, I finally left the hospital. Sleepy, tired, and hungry, I stumbled back to the Phi Chi house to try to catch some sleep. Along the way, I met Oscar and Walter on their way to the hospital. I told them about the patient of the night as we passed. They were moving into the day as I was moving out of the night.

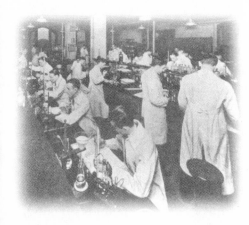

22

JUST A
MATTER
OF PRIDE

Senior medical students are permitted to work in certain approved clinical settings at night and on weekends.

Comments of the Dean
Fall 1954

THE SENIOR YEAR CAME, AND WE SCATTERED AS A CLASS. Nearly everyone had a part-time job at night and on weekends in the senior year. Given our very small groups in the short clinic rotations of the senior year, and our night and weekend jobs, we saw each other less and less. Friday night dinners at the Phi Chi house had come to an end. We had heard the last of Oscar's mother's letters. There were no more imitations of faculty to come from Wally, who was now a surgical intern at Vanderbilt. No more awards for the horniest medical student of the week. It was time for the family to scatter. At the end of the year, all of us would be moving to internships at sites still unknown. The senior year was preparatory for our final separations.

Senior jobs were nearly universal for the students in our class. Most of the jobs were centered around taking admission histories and transcribing orders from private physicians—so called externships. Jean externed at Saint Thomas Hospital, as did several other classmates. Several classmates were externs at night at the huge Central State Insane Asylum, which housed more than two thousand involuntarily

159

committed patients. Such confinement was then allowed by law. Oscar was in-house doctor at one of the children's homes. Three classmates covered sick call at the state penitentiary. Others provided in-house night coverage at the area's tuberculosis sanatorium.

Five of us had accepted the job of giving anesthesia to obstetrical cases at night. We had to take a two-month course in the summer to prepare ourselves. We lived in an old house immediately behind the hospital with the surgical house staff and took call every fifth night. The only pay any of us received was free room, board, and laundry. The food was unlimited, and I gained nearly twenty pounds thinking, stupidly, that the more I ate, the more I was being paid.

Visiting each other's workplaces became a favorite pastime. I spent time with classmates at the penitentiary, the state insane asylum, and the tuberculosis sanatorium. But my favorite visits were those with Hank at a small hospital across town.

Hank had the job with the most responsibility. He ran the emergency room at night and on weekends for the small private hospital. Two other classmates worked there in the ER all night every third night and weekends. Most of the patients had problems that were not serious, life-threatening emergencies. It was more of a night clinic to cover the practice of the private physicians than an ER.

I spent several nights there through the year watching Hank do his job and helping out when he got overloaded. It was fun but more than I would have taken on, given our level of inexperience. Hank felt otherwise. Like all surgeons, Hank was fearless. He had telephone backup from one of the private physicians, whom he could call at any time for help, yet Hank almost never called the man. It was a matter of pride.

One night, this pride nearly tripped him up. A small boy and his father were sitting in the small treatment room when Hank and I walked in. Hank stuck out his hand and introduced himself as "Dr. Meiers." He looked like he had been saying it for twenty years. I was impressed.

The boy had fallen down roller-skating and injured his right wrist. He was sitting in his father's lap with tear-stained streaks down his dirty face. The father was in coveralls coated in grease, obviously a mechanic of some sort. When he stood, he eased the boy to his feet, reached out and shook Hank's hand. The man looked like a tight end on some pro football team. He was at least six feet, five inches, and weighed more than Hank and me together.

Hank mumbled, "This Dr. Meador. He's working with me tonight."

The father extended his hand. It looked like a baseball mitt. "Good to know you," the father said.

Hank ordered an X-ray of the hand, wrist, and elbow. He told me he did this so he wouldn't miss any higher fractures. I have never had anyone tell us to X-ray the joint above an injury. Hank just made it up.

The X-rays showed a Colles's fracture of the right head of the radius. This is the classic fracture that occurs when falling on extended hands. The wrist snaps back and breaks the bone just above the wrist.

The boy cried when Hank told him he had a broken bone.

We retreated into the private doctor's office. Every chair and tabletop was filled with scattered medical journals. The shelves were filled with books, some dating back to the early 1900s. There was a lab coat thrown over a chair. The desk was covered in drug samples and literature left by the drug detail men. A small X-ray viewing box was on the wall over a small sink. Hank popped the film onto the viewer and pointed out the fine fracture line to me. On side view the radius appeared bent slightly backward. You could visualize the nature of the injury by seeing the backward displacement of the wrist on impact.

"Let's see what the books say to do here," Hank said as he scanned an orthopedic book. He read rapidly to himself, slammed the book shut, and said, "No problem. Let's go cast the arm."

"You ever do this before?" I asked.

"Nope," Hank answered over his shoulder.

"Don't you think you should call the surgeon?" I asked, nervous that Hank was moving into some forbidden zone. I had no idea how to put on a cast. Hank didn't answer me.

Hank wrapped the boy's arm in soft gauze. Then he rolled out the wet plaster gauze and wrapped it around the boy's hand and wrist, extending the wet plaster all the way to the elbow. Then he smoothed the plaster, and in a few minutes he had put on a very professional looking cast. He patted the boy on the head, told the father to look at the fingers and check for feeling every three to four hours, and to come back if the hand got blue or the fingers numb. The man was profuse with thanks and left. Hank and I resumed tending to the modest stream of patients with colds or sore throats or small lacerations and abrasions.

In less than half an hour, I heard a loud voice coming from the waiting room. The voice got closer, and soon the boy's father turned the corner. Gone was the thankful, respectful man we had sent on his way. This man was furious. "Where is that young doctor?" he shouted. "I want to see him . . . NOW!"

Hank stuck his head out of an exam room. The man stalked up to Hank's face and stuck a white plaster cast right into it. "What kind of sloppy work is this?! Boy gets out my truck at home. The whole cast falls off. Right there! Falls off."

Hank didn't hesitate. Without backing away from the father one bit, and even looking slightly irritated, he said simply: "Now exactly how was your son holding his arm? I want to know that before we talk."

The man stopped, hesitated, and said, "Uh, well, like this I guess." He held his arm down by his side imitating how he thought the son did.

"See," Hank said in a loud voice, shaking his head, "I thought that's what happened." Hank actually looked frustrated. "I told you to have him keep that arm in that sling. You can't go around dangling a new cast. Now I've got to put the dern cast back on."

The man was all apologies. He followed Hank to the treatment room and kept saying how sorry he was, and how he was sorry to put Hank to all that trouble.

Hank suddenly turned and, with the straightest possible face, said, "It won't be any trouble at all. I was just a little upset."

Although Hank was wrong to have moved into medical territory he did not know, I knew at another level that Hank was a natural surgeon.

No matter how bad or desperate or how scary a situation was, Hank had the one quality required of all surgeons in emergencies— imperturbability.

After he finished putting on the new cast, Hank slid into the office and collapsed on the sofa. Hank vowed that was his one and only cast until he had orthopedic training. "Good golly," he said. "Can you believe the first cast I ever put on fell off? Fell right off. I was making sure I didn't get it on too tight. I thought that man was going to whip my ass. Don't you tell Oscar or Jean or anybody about this."

"Hank, I just can't wait." I laughed and sat down next to him. Hank was a constant source of great stories for the lounge.

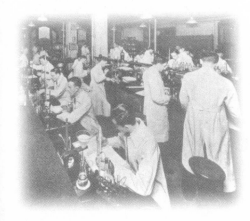

23

THE
LAST CHAPTER

Requirements for Graduation. — The candidate for the degree of Doctor of Medicine must have achieved the age of 21 years and be of good moral character. They must spend at least 4 years of study as matriculated medical students, the last 2 of which must have been in this school. They must have satisfactorily completed all prescribed examinations and be free of indebtedness to the University. At the end of the 4th year every student who has fulfilled these requirements will be recommended for the degree of Doctor of Medicine.

Catalogue for 1954–1955
School of Medicine
Vanderbilt University

THE SENIOR YEAR WOUND DOWN AND FINALLY CAME TO its end. Our last year of school was as unstressful as the first three years were overloaded with stress. I wondered if it was designed that way on purpose. Maybe it was a way of resting us up for the deadliest of all stressful years—internship.

There was no night call in any of the courses or rotations. We rotated from one clinic to another, a kind of cafeteria of the specialties then in existence. We usually spent about two weeks in each clinic getting a taste of the clinical problems of that specialty. Most of these clinics met only once a week. If a patient had problems involving several organs, it could take a month or two to go from one clinic to another to get all of the outpatient consultations. Someone once overheard a social worker ask a man what kind of work he did for a living. He answered, "Ma'am, you can't hold down a full-time job and 'tend the university clinics."

Some afternoons, Oscar, Jean, Hank, and I played golf. Our evenings were mostly free. To some extent we rejoined the outside world. The Korean War, its details little-known to us, had ended. We began to date again. We saw movies and played poker on Wednesday nights at the Phi Chi house. We had time to catch up on our reading, nearly impossible during most of the third year. It was like a wonderful needed rest cure after a protracted illness.

I had not seen Wally for several months. He had stayed on after graduation as a surgical intern, and had been out at the VA Hospital. I barely recognized him. He was hollow-eyed and had lost at least twenty pounds. He looked like one of those soldiers from World War II movies who had escaped from a Japanese prisoner of war camp.

"Just you wait. Just wait," Wally said as we sat down to have a Coke in the cafeteria. "If you thought Jungle Jim was bad, or if you go around thinking Shapiro was tough, try interning. Hell, I haven't slept in weeks. I'm way past spazzed. I'm beat." Wally went on and on, expanding on his fatigue and torment. But again, as always, there was that lurking reality beneath Wally's bluster.

Medical school then and now prepares one for only one thing—the next step on the educational path toward becoming a real doctor— internship. Beginning the search for an internship became our highest priority. My first turn was toward Alabama, my native state. In 1954, Tinsley Harrison had already become a legend. His textbook, *Principles of Internal Medicine*, was becoming the new national standard, and he had become the chairman of medicine at the University of Alabama in Birmingham. I was attracted to him and his way of thinking. I already knew I wanted to follow a career in academic medicine.

When I came into Dr. Harrison's office, he stood, came around the desk, and shook my hand. He exuded high energy and spoke in a clipped Southern accent that I have come to call "Southern emphatic." Although that accent is disappearing, you may still hear it in older Southerners who were educated in the north. He got right to the point.

"I would love to have you here. But I am not going to offer you a place. You wrote that you are interested in academic medicine. Go east. Get well trained. Go to Boston, New York, Hopkins. Come back and be on my faculty. I am not ready to offer you what you can get in the East." He stood and headed me toward the door.

He paused just before he shook my hand. "Remember this. Always put the person before the institution. If something is good for the institution, but bad for the person, don't do it. If it is good for the person AND good for the institution, then do it. It would be good for us to have you here. It would not be good for you. Go east." He shook my hand and said good-bye. I did not see him again until I joined his faculty eight years later.

Just before the first trimester, in August of 1954, Hank, two other classmates, and I headed east for a week's trip. We went by train to New York and Boston, which required changes in Atlanta, Washington, and New York. Hank was looking at surgical programs, and I was visiting medical departments. I had my heart set on Bellevue, where I knew I would see the greatest variety of clinical problems.

In Boston, I had interviews at the Mass General, Peter Bent Brigham, and the Harvard service at Boston City. In New York, I was scheduled for interviews at Columbia Presbyterian on the Upper West Side, Cornell's New York Hospital on the Upper East Side, and the Cornell service at Bellevue on the Lower East Side. I quickly learned to use the subway.

Bellevue had the reputation of being the toughest internship in existence. Being tough and taking on huge loads was part of the desired game in those days for most of us. Machismo to the maximum. That's what I thought I wanted until I visited Bellevue.

I spent the morning with the house staff and was scheduled to have my interview with the chief of the service just before noon. My first look at the house officers began to turn my mind. Their white coats had turned into a filthy dull gray, with streaks and smudges of black and blood here and there. Three of them fell asleep during morning report. None of them had shaved.

On walking rounds they described their daily routine not only of drawing all the bloods, but taking the specimens to the lab and doing the lab work, chemistries and all. Then they rushed back so they could wheel the patients going for X-rays down to radiology only in time to rush back to the ward to work up the next four or five daily admissions, only to begin the process all over. Interns at Bellevue did it all, single-handed. There was no support staff other than a nurse or two. Interns and nurses—that was it.

To cap it all, they told me they had become short-handed. One resident and one intern were out with open tuberculosis, having acquired it on the service. An occasional case was not at all unusual for any teaching hospital in those days, but two in one year was extreme.

My initial enthusiasm for Bellevue was falling minute by minute. I wanted to leave, but I had the interview scheduled, so I waited. I walked into the chief's office. He was a big name in academic circles, having served as president of the Old Turks the year before. Just as I sat down, all the pretense I had mustered vanished. Before I knew it, I could hear myself telling him that I had decided to withdraw my name from consideration for an internship at Bellevue. I said something about not wanting to waste his time and some other mutterings as I stood and headed for the door. His eyes followed me to the door as I backed out of the room. He didn't say one word. He had the most incredulous expression on his face as he stood.

When I got to the street outside, I inhaled deep breaths of relief. I walked around to a high ridge of concrete and looked out on the East River below and to Brooklyn on the opposite bank. I felt like I had escaped from Devil's Island. If you ever see a doctor who trained at Bellevue, stand and take off your hat and know that you are in the presence of a member of the French Foreign Legion of medicine—the toughest of the tough. They will have seen and done everything, and that more than once. Every conceivable disease of every derelict and mistreated soul pours in there from all over the City of New York. They see it all. I envied that opportunity, to see that wide a spectrum of disease, but I knew I did not have the stamina or will to take on a Bellevue internship.

I went on to interviews at Columbia Presbyterian and Cornell's New York Hospital. I stood in the solarium on the ninth floor of Presbyterian Hospital when I went on rounds with Dr. Robert Loeb, chairman of medicine. As I looked back downtown, I could see it all. Central Park was off to the left. The Hudson River sparkled beneath on the right, with all of Manhattan tapering into the Battery in the hazy distance. This was where I wanted to be.

In mid-March we would learn where we would do our internships and most likely spend the next several years of residency; it was, in all likelihood, where we would settle and practice or do research and teach.

There are only a few days in any life where one day makes such an enormous difference—the day we are born, the day we get married, the day a son or daughter is born, and most certainly the day we die. I would put the day of the internship match at that level of importance. I thought it strange, and still do, how much fate and destiny hangs on a single day. All over the country, senior medical students open envelopes on the same day in mid-March and literally read their fate on a piece of paper. The imagined life that might have happened in one location vanishes into the second- or third-choice location for internship, sometimes in a very different city or section of the country. In a flash, one sees the next several years come into focus.

The letter in my envelope was from Dr. Robert Loeb, chairman and chief of medicine at Columbia Presbyterian Hospital in New York. It said he was glad to offer me an invitation to serve as a medical intern on his service. I flopped into the nearest chair. My breath was rapid. The hair on my arms and neck bristled. I had gotten what I wanted most. I would be in New York—the Big Apple. I wanted to yell and jump and run. Hank came up to me grinning. He got his first choice too—surgery at Barnes and Washington University. Jean, Oscar, and Ben would stay at Vanderbilt. Walter would go to the Harvard medical service at Boston City. All of us got our first choices. I heard that all of our class got their first choices also.

After March there wasn't much attention left for school. We all made plans for our moves and mostly partied.

Graduation that year had to be moved into Memorial Gym from the lawn because of rain. Dean Rusk, later to be secretary of state under Presidents Kennedy and Johnson, was the commencement speaker. I don't remember a single word he said, not even his topic. My mind was racing from one face to the next as I looked back at the audience from our seats on the gym floor. My family was there, as were the families of Oscar, Hank, Jean, Walter, and Ben. But then the faces of the faculty came into focus. Jungle Jim Ward from Anatomy; Meng from Physiology; and Meneely from the VA; then Shapiro from Pathology; Hartman and Kampmeier and Newman. Nearly the entire faculty was there. Dean John Youmans handed me my diploma, and I became Doctor Meador.

Now I would start all over again—freshman to senior to freshman to senior to freshman—a repeating cycle that would continue for another seven years of internship, then residency, then Army medical corps, back to residency and fellowship, then junior member of a practice group, and finally junior faculty at Alabama with Dr. Tinsley Harrison.

I have heard some doctors say that what they learned in medical school bears little resemblance to what they do on a day-to-day basis in their practice. They point to the rapid rate of change in scientific and medical knowledge and the explosion of technology that surrounds us. While those advances have occurred, and while we know much more about the workings of disease and health, I do not have those same views.

The faculty and the patients of the Vanderbilt University School of Medicine at mid-twentieth century taught me those fundamentals of caring for patients that are timeless. They were true then, and they will remain true. Foremost on this list is the ability to listen to a patient as a fellow human being, with the same feelings, troubles, problems, and diseases as all of us may have. But beyond listening Vanderbilt taught me to place the disease of the patient in the setting and story that is unique for the life of that particular and specific patient.

"It is as important to know the patient with the disease as it is to know the disease." I don't remember which professor first said that. Diseases change and come and go. Technology follows science and knowledge, and it too comes and goes. Human nature and spirit do not come and go. The fundamentals of what I learned at Vanderbilt with my classmates in the class of '55 have endured and have only enhanced the incredible advances in science and technology of the past fifty years.

Epilogue

An attempt is also made to interest the student in the relation of disease and injury to society and to awaken in him a consciousness of his broader obligations to his community and to its social organization.

> Catalogue for 1951–1952
> School of Medicine
> Vanderbilt University

THE MID-TWENTIETH CENTURY FOLLOWING WORLD WAR II was a time of transition. These stories of classmates and professors and patients are from a medical school that was removed from the larger world. We were cloistered from the major events of the day—the Korean War and the emerging Cold War with the U.S.S.R., with its threat of nuclear devastation. We lived in the Deep South, and knew only its completely segregated worlds of black and white. Martin Luther King Jr. was just finishing graduate school, and *Brown* vs. *the Board of Education* was before the U.S. Supreme Court. There were no black medical students and no black faculty in the medical school. There was one ward in the hospital for black patients. There were only two women in the class of 1955.

The faculty of the School of Medicine numbered 382 in the 1951–1952 catalogue. Of that, 302 were in private practice and gave their time with no pay. There were only 80 full-time members. Many of those also maintained private practices to supplement their incomes.

In 1951, as these stories show, women had not yet entered medicine in any large numbers. There were only fifteen women on the faculty. There was an average of only two women in each class. Although they were few in number, three of the women faculty members played important and formative roles in our education.

Dr. Mary Gray single-handedly taught the course in Histology. She was a breath of wonderful perfume and enlightenment, in a world then filled with formalin.

Dr. Ann Minot, a biochemist of some note, ran the central chemistry laboratory. Dr. Minot and her associate, Helen Frank, not only made the measurements, they followed the patients carefully. They knew the clinical problems of the patients and the reasons for their admissions. They often called to tell us that a BUN had gone up or that one of the liver function tests had become abnormal or that some other measurement had changed. Dr. Minot also taught us acid/base and fluid and electrolyte management. Both women were forces to be reckoned with, especially if we messed up a specimen or put blood in the wrong tube.

Dr. Mildred Stahlman, then a junior member of the faculty, taught us care of the newborn. Millie, as we called her, went on to a very distinguished career in her work in understanding and maintaining the immature lung of the premature infant. She was the first physician ever to mechanically ventilate an infant. That contribution alone has saved hundreds of thousands of premature infants. Millie Stahlman was one of the leading creators of the new field of neonatology.

In 1951, our entering class had numbered fifty-two, the usual class size of that time. By the end of the second year, the class stood at forty-four. Seven had failed or been asked to withdraw, and one was killed in an automobile accident. Three classmates transferred into the third year from the two-year medical schools then in existence, making a total of forty-seven graduating seniors in the class of 1955.

The class scattered to twenty-two locations for internships and residencies. The ultimate careers of the forty-seven classmates fell into the following specialties:

General surgeons	5
Neurosurgeons	4
Thoracic surgeons	2
Cardiac surgeons	3
Ophthalmologists	2
Orthopedic surgeons	2
Urological surgeons	3
Obstetricians and Gynecologists	2
Internists/Medical Specialists	8
Radiologists	1
Pediatricians	8
Pathologists	3
Psychiatrists	3
Neurologists	1

Nearly half of the class went on to full-time or part-time academic careers. As of 2002, eight of the forty-seven classmates have died.

Hank (Henry Meiers) went to Saint Louis for an internship and residency in surgery at Barnes Hospital of Washington University. After service in the Army, he lived out his life as a distinguished general surgeon in Kentucky. From time to time, I saw patients he referred to me for medical consultations before he died several years ago.

Jean (Cortner) spent one year in pediatrics at Vanderbilt, and then did his residency at the Babies' Hospital at Columbia Presbyterian Hospital in New York City, returning to Vanderbilt as chief resident. Following a two-year Army tour in Paris, Jean trained extensively in biochemical genetics, first at Rockefeller Institute and later as a special fellow at the Galton Laboratory in London. Jean went on to be a distinguished chairman of pediatrics at two universities. After serving as chief of pediatrics at Roswell Park Memorial Institute, he became chairman of pediatrics at the State University of New York at Buffalo and pediatrician-in-chief at the Children's Hospital of Buffalo for seven years. He then became chairman of pediatrics at the University of Pennsylvania and physician-in-chief of the Children's Hospital of

Philadelphia. In 1999 he was honored with the creation of the Jean Cortner Endowed Chair of Pediatrics at the Children's Hospital of Philadelphia. Jean and his wife, Jeanne, split their time between Jackson Hole, Wyoming, and Philadelphia.

After a year in pediatrics at Vanderbilt, Ben (Richard Benjamin Moore) switched to urological surgery. He did his residency in urology at the University of Tennessee. Following his residency, he did a fellowship in urological pathology at the Armed Forces Institute of Pathology. After service in the Navy, he became an outstanding urologist, practicing in the Miami/Palm Beach area of Florida. He and his wife, Connie, now live in southern Florida and North Carolina.

After a year in medicine at Vanderbilt, Oscar (Crofford) spent several years in biochemistry in Switzerland, and then returned to Vanderbilt, where he became professor of medicine and the first director of the N.I.H.–funded Diabetes Research and Training Center. Oscar, the most distinguished and accomplished scientist of our class, led the entire national effort, from conception to funding to implementation to completion, in the monumental study of the controlled treatment of diabetes mellitus. His multicenter study showed, conclusively and for the first time, that control of blood glucose levels reduces the vascular complications of diabetes mellitus.

Oscar received many awards and recognitions for his monumental contributions to the understanding and treatment of diabetes mellitus. Among these awards were the Lily Award in 1970, the Banting Medal of the American Diabetes Association in 1982, and the Novo Award of the Irish Endocrine Society in 1994. He received the Charles H. Best Award twice, first in 1976, and again in 1994. In 1996, the University of Toronto conferred the Doctor of Science, *honoris causa*, on the seventy-fifth anniversary of the discovery of insulin by Banting and Best at the University in 1921. In 1999, he was awarded the Novartis Award as the first recipient of that award for Lifetime Achievement. Oscar and his wife, Jane, live on his beloved farm in Arkansas, where they raise cows.

Wally (Wallace Faulk) completed his general surgical training at Vanderbilt. He then trained for four years in the department of hthalmology at the University of Iowa. Following a stint in the Navy, he practiced ophthalmology in Nashville, where he still lives.

Walter (Puckett) trained at the Harvard medical service at Boston City Hospital, Boston's equivalent of Bellevue. Following a stint in the Navy in the Underwater Demolition Force (forerunner of the Navy SEALS), he returned to Vanderbilt. He completed his training as a fellow in cardiology at Vanderbilt, and practiced and taught cardiology in Chattanooga, Tennessee.

I returned to Vanderbilt in 1973, to join the full-time faculty and to establish the Vanderbilt teaching service at Saint Thomas Hospital. In addition to teaching, I had a busy private and referral practice. It was my great privilege to serve as personal physician for a number of the older faculty, including Dean John Youmans, Dr. Rudolph Kampmeier, Dr. James "Jungle Jim" Ward, Dr. Ann Minot, and Helen Frank. I became especially close to Dr. John Shapiro, with whom I shared and discussed many of the stories in this book.

About the Author

CLIFTON K. MEADOR GRADUATED FROM VANDERBILT University School of Medicine in 1955, sharing the Founder's Medal for top scholastic honors with a classmate. Dr. Meador directed the N.I.H. Clinical Research Center at the University of Alabama in Birmingham for six years, advanced to professor of medicine, and served as dean of the School of Medicine at the university from 1968 to 1973.

In 1973 Dr. Meador returned to Vanderbilt to join the full-time faculty as professor of medicine and to establish the Vanderbilt teaching service in medicine at Saint Thomas Hospital. Dr. Meador also served as chief medical officer of the hospital until 1998, when he became the executive director of the newly formed Meharry-Vanderbilt Alliance. He is now professor of medicine at both medical schools and continues to direct the programs of the alliance.

Dr. Meador has published extensively in the medical literature; he is perhaps best known for "The Art and Science of Nondisease" and "The Last Well Person," both published in the New England Journal of Medicine, and "A Lament for Invalids," published in the Journal of the American Medical Association. The articles are satiric treatments of the excesses of medical practice. He is the author of seven books, including the bestseller *A Little Book of Doctors' Rules*.

Dr. Meador lives in Nashville, Tennessee, with his wife, Kathleen. He has seven children and seven grandchildren.